Your premature baby

0–5 years

Nikki Bradford

*photographs by
Sandra Lousada*

FRANCES LINCOLN

Tommy's Campaign benefits from the sale of this book.
Tommy's Campaign, the national pregnancy research charity, funds a nationwide programme of research into miscarriage, stillbirth and premature birth and provides information to parents and midwives on pregnancy issues.

Frances Lincoln Ltd
4 Torriano Mews
Torriano Avenue
London NW5 2RZ

Your Premature Baby: 0–5 Years
Copyright © Frances Lincoln Limited 2000
Text copyright © Nikki Bradford 2000
Photographs copyright © Sandra Lousada 2000,
except for those listed on page 208
Foreword copyright © Ian Fergusson 2000

First Frances Lincoln edition: 2000

British Library Cataloguing in Publication data
A catalogue record for this book is available from the British Library.

ISBN 0 7112 1614 2

Printed in Singapore

This book is intended to be a guide for parents who wish to understand more about their baby's condition and is not intended to replace the advice of a medical practitioner. Medical advice should always be sought before undertaking any form of treatment and it should be noted that advances in medical science may result in information contained in this book becoming out of date.

2 4 6 8 9 7 5 3 1

contents

We have adopted the convention of calling the baby 'he' in one chapter, 'she' in the next.

foreword

Hospitals are frightening places. Intensive Care Units are more frightening, and Special Care Baby Units and Neonatal Intensive Care Units, probably the most frightening.

Frightened parents and relatives can find it hard to cope with all the stresses that surround premature birth and especially the extreme pressures that are the inevitable consequences of watching your own tiny baby fighting for survival in a stark technological environment.

Explanations from the medical staff may of necessity be guarded and lack clarity. Pressures of work may limit the comfort and support given to parents. Fear and reticence may inhibit the parents from asking questions. Stress and anxiety may make it difficult to absorb and rationalize the answers that are given.

This book sponsored by Tommy's Campaign is designed to alleviate some of these worries. It aims to provide some of the background to prematurity and poor fetal growth in the womb. It explains how special care baby units function – and it suggests ways in which parents can best help their babies through this very difficult chapter in life.

The book is written in easily understood language, decoding medical jargon and opening up the way to the best possible care of premature babies by encouraging team work between the parents and the hospital staff.

It offers comfort, support and invaluable knowledge to the very many new mothers and fathers facing the challenge of a premature baby. It will also be highly informative reading for the staff of premature baby units.

Tommy's Campaign is a charity that exists to promote research and understanding into the causes and prevention of prematurity. We work unceasingly to reduce the incidence of premature births, but while it still exists we hope that this book may provide a most valuable source of information and encouragement.

Ian Fergusson FRCS FRCOG
Consultant Obstetrician and Gynaecologist, St Thomas' Hospital, London
Chairman, Tommy's Campaign

author's acknowledgments

This book would not have been possible without the following people, who gave so generously of their time, advice, experience and expertise.

Very special thanks to:

Dr Anthony Michael Kaiser, Consultant Neonatologist at St Thomas' Hospital, London, for his invaluable help, tireless encouragement and advice on the sections about premature babies' possible medical problems and what can be done about them. He read much of the manuscript standing up on the tube on his way home after long, hot, late days and nights at the SCBU.

And to:

Andrew Whitelaw, Professor of Neonatal Medicine at the University of Bristol, Southmead Hospital, Neil Marlow, Professor of Neonatal Medicine at Nottingham University, and Ros Jones, Consultant Neonatologist, Wrexham Park Hospital, Slough, for their help and suggestions on the chapter on the outcome for premature babies as they grow up.

Professor Phillip Bennett, Imperial College School of Medicine, London, for his help with the section on possible causes of premature labour.

Professor Neil McIntosh, neonatologist and Professor of Child Life & Health at the University of Edinburgh, for his help in connection with his work on cerebral palsy and premature babies.

Dr Jeanine Young, at the time of writing developmental care expert, author and Research Midwife at the Department of Child Health, Bristol, for her support and advice on all the developmental care issues, including positioning and premature babies' communication.

Geoffrey Chamberlain, Professor Emeritus at the Singleton Hospital, Swansea, and immediate past President of the Royal College of Obstetricians & Gynaecologists, for his suggestions for the section on possible causes of prematurity.

Simon Roth, Consultant Paediatrician at Barnet Hospital, London, for help with the section on paediatric osteopathy.

Susan Bewley, Consultant Obstetrician at St Thomas' Hospital, London, for her invaluable suggestions and feedback for the section on possible causes of prematurity.

Tilly Padden, at the time of writing neonatal nursing sister, researcher, midwife and Senior Lecturer in Midwifery Studies at the University of Lancashire, for all her help with the chapter on *You and your family*.

Sandra Lang, Consultant in Infant Feeding to UNICEF and the WHO, specialist in breast-feeding/cup-feeding of premature babies, for her advice on feeding.

Lisa Hollis, Community Liaison Neonatal Sister at Kingston Hospital NHS Trust, for invaluable guidance on and contributions to the chapters on *How little you are* and *Time to go home*.

Bridgette Riley, Family Care Sister at Derby City General Hospital, and Head of the Neonatal Nurses Association's Special Interest Group of Community Neonatal Sisters for her help with *You and your family* and *Time to go home*.

Chrissie Israel, Research Sister, and Parent-Baby Interaction Advisor at Southmead Hospital, Bristol NHS Trust, for her help with *You and your family*.

Joan Ritchie, neonatal nursing sister at Southmead Hospital, Bristol NHS Trust, for her advice on feeding.

Alree Hunt, neonatal nursing sister at St Thomas' Hospital, London, for all her input into the chapter on how being born early may affect your baby.

Kathy Sleath, neonatal nursing practitioner of the Hammersmith Hospital, London, for her pioneering work with kangaroo care in the UK, and her help with this section of the book.

Monica Yonge, neonatal sister at Kingston Hospital NHS Trust, for her help.

Anna Collett, neonatal senior staff nurse and co-ordinator of the breast-milk bank at Kingston Hospital NHS Trust, for her suggestions on feeding.

Angela Newton, neonatal sister at the Starlight Unit, Barnet Hospital, London, and **Julie Honeychurch**, senior neonatal nurse and former sister at Southmead Hospital, Bristol, for their invaluable advice on positioning premature babies.

Janet Venn, neonatal sister at Musgrave Park Hospital (at the Taunton and Somerset NHS Trust), for her advice on therapeutic touch, colour therapy and massage for premature babies.

Jenni Thomas, Founder-Director of The Child Bereavement Trust, and Bereavement Counsellor at Wycombe General Hospital, for all her help and support with the chapter on grieving and the loss of a baby.

Clare Delpech, Founder-Director of the Association for Post-Natal Illness, for her help with the section on post-natal depression.

Stuart Korf, Founder and Director of the registered charity The Children's Osteopathic Clinic in London, and Consultant Paediatric Osteopath **Susie Booth**, also of the COC, for their advice on how specialist paediatric osteopathy can be used to help and support premature babies – and the toddlers and children they become.

Philip Beech, osteopath/acupuncturist; and Senior Examiner/Lecturer at both the British School of Osteopathy and at the College of Naturopathy & Osteopathy, for information and practical suggestions for the chapter on *You and your family*.

Pauline Woods, Co-ordinator of Kingston Hospital NHS Trust's charity Born Too Soon, for all her kindness, enthusiasm and invaluable help with many different aspects of this book.

Dr Sarah Levine, Medical Officer at the Foundation for the Study of Infant Deaths.

BLISS, the premature baby parents' support charity, for their help with the chapter on *What happens now?* and for some immensely helpful suggestions as to which experts to approach for other chapters.

The Neonatal Nurses Association for very kindly putting us in touch with some of their specialist members.

Mark Hollinsworth, Researcher at the Information and Statistics Division (Scotland) Common Services Agency for the National Health Service for freely donating his time to track down various hard-to-find statistics in several different chapters.

All the SCBU nursing staff at St Thomas' Hospital, London; at **Kingston Hospital NHS Trust**, Surrey, and at **Southmead Hospital**, Bristol: for their time, patience and suggestions on several chapters.

Ruth Hudson of The Health Visitors' Association, for her advice on normal developmental checks for babies, toddlers and children.

And in America:

Professor Peter Nathanielz, New York, for his encouragement and suggestions right at the beginning of this project.

Professor John McGregor, Head of Obstetrics & Gynaecology at Colorado University, for his advice and vision regarding the chapter on possible causes of premature labour.

And, very importantly, to the many dozens of parents of premature babies, who helped with advice and suggestions based on their hard-won experience.

Special thanks to:

The **Born Too Soon Parents Support Group** in Kingston, based at Wellcare House, and **Pauline Woods**, who took such time and trouble to introduce us; **Caroline and Trefor Hughes-Jenkins**, whose triplets, Tom, Ben and Megan, were born at 29 weeks; **Ashleigh and Mike**, whose daughter, Scarlett, was born at 31 weeks; **Louise Fulgoni**, whose daughter, Gabrielle, was born at 24 weeks; **Meera**, whose son, Rohan, was born at 26 weeks; and **Catherine Gibson**, whose son, Mark, was born at 31 weeks. Grateful thanks and admiration also to **Jo and Robert Robinson** from Nottingham whose son, Gregor, was born at 29 weeks and to **Bettina and Clive Radford** from Liverpool whose twin girls, Susanna and Madeline, were born at 33 weeks.

Your premature baby may not look like the one in the baby milk adverts: in fact it's likely that he will temporarily look very different – sometimes disturbingly so, especially if he is very premature. He will also differ from a baby born at full term in the things he can and cannot do for himself and how much help and medical support he may need for a while. These differences between the way your baby looks now and the mental image you had of the baby you'd hoped for may be upsetting, surprising or difficult to come to grips with, but it can help if you know roughly what to expect and the reasons for the differences. This chapter covers what babies of different degrees of prematurity may look like and what they may possibly be able to do or handle.

Born at 26 weeks: 'I couldn't believe anything this tiny could survive. He was so small and skinny and looked like even a light touch would bruise him.'

What does that word mean?

Medical staff may use terms that you have not heard before or whose technical meaning is unfamiliar:

Premature/preterm/prem baby:
a baby who has been born before spending 37 weeks in the womb.

Gestational age (GA):
the amount of time your baby has spent in your womb. If he is 25 weeks gestational age he has spent 25 weeks growing inside you. This means he is about 15 weeks early, as most babies arrive between 38 and 41 weeks GA.

Extremely premature:
born having spent 24 to 28 weeks in the womb.

Very premature:
born having spent 29 to 34 weeks in the womb.

Moderately premature:
born having spent 35 to 37 weeks in the womb.

Low birthweight baby:
a baby who weighs less than 2,500g (5½lb) at birth. Most premature babies are also low birthweight. However, the two terms do not mean the same thing, because some babies can spend all 40 weeks in the womb, but still be smaller than usual when they arrive. (See also **Birthweight** on page 14.)

Very or extremely low birthweight baby:
a baby born weighing less than 1,361g (3lb).

Term baby:
a baby who has spent the full amount of time developing in the womb – between 38 and 41 weeks.

Viability limit:
how early a premature baby can be born and still live. Different hospitals have slightly different limits for the age at which they feel a premature baby can be helped. Although a very few babies have survived after being born at 22 weeks, viability limits usually fall somewhere between 23 and 25 weeks.

Nine out of ten premature babies survive and go home with their parents

Worrying though it is to see this tiny, vulnerable little being, your baby *will* change, develop, grow and mature – often more quickly than you imagined was possible when he began his life in such a fragile state.

'Such a tiny scrap of humanity, linked up to all those wires and dwarfed by machines. She didn't seem like a baby, more a half-human little animal, an essential component in a complicated life-support machine.'

Pete, father of Emma, born at 27 weeks

Factors affecting what your baby can do

These include:

* Your baby's own particular personality and temperament

* His own special strengths and weaknesses

* How well he is and has been

* Any operations he has had

* Any medicines he is having

* How he is being cared for

* If and how he is being supported by technology – a baby on a ventilator can cope with far less than a baby receiving oxygen via a small nasal prong

* Whether he has recently had any tests (such as X-rays) or invasive procedures (such as regular clearing of his artificial breathing tube) that may have distressed or tired him

Birthweight

A baby's weight at birth also makes a difference to what he can do and cope with. A baby born at, say, 32 weeks, might have the typical birthweight of a baby born much earlier – say at 28 weeks. In this case birthweight can be a better guide to how he may cope than gestational age.

Low birthweight can (though does not always) mean that there were problems with development in the womb, and your baby may show characteristics of or share problems with a more premature baby.

YOUR BABY'S PERSONAL COPING TIMETABLE

The information in this chapter is only a very general guide to what a premature baby looks like, can do or can cope with, at a particular age. Babies are individuals from the moment they are born, no matter how early they arrive. What they can manage and when varies a great deal from baby to baby – even between those of the same gestational age – and depends on many different factors.

There are variations, too, within age groups. For instance, even though babies of 24 and 28 weeks are considered together as 'extremely premature', differences also depend on exactly how many weeks early they are. There is an enormous difference between what an unwell premature baby of 25 weeks GA can do and cope with, and what a relatively well 28-week premature baby can manage.

IF YOUR BABY IS BORN AT 24 to 28 WEEKS

If your baby is 16 to 12 weeks early he is likely to weigh 454g–1,600g (1–3½lb). He will be about 25–33cm (10–13in) long, and spend most of the time – at least 80 per cent of his day – trying to sleep.

How your baby may look

He will have a relatively large head – it is not yet in proportion with his body – and some downy hair on his face and body. This is called lanugo and is normal for the stage your baby had reached in your womb. It appeared at 17–20 weeks and will disappear quite naturally at around the time your baby would have been born; hair on his back may rub off sooner, because he is lying on it.

He will probably seem very thin and fragile to you. As the fatty layer under the skin has not yet had time to build up, his skin will seem transparent: you can clearly see the delicate pattern of blood vessels threading their way across his body. His skin tone will usually be darkish red, at first, because his circulation may not be very good yet, and his blood may not contain enough oxygen. Your baby's skin may also look 'waxy', but this effect will disappear as he matures. He may have some bruising on his skin, which is very sensitive to touch (even a monitor lead lying in the same place for a time can cause bruising).

Your baby's eyes may still be fused shut, like a new-born kitten's. All babies have their eyes shut from about ten womb-weeks to around week 26, when their eyes open naturally. When his eyes are shut, his eyeballs may bulge a little against their lids, and he may not yet have eyelashes. His ears are soft and flexible: if they are bent back they will not be able to spring back into position as the cartilage in them has not yet formed firmly enough. He has the beginning delicate buds of fingernails and toenails, and perfectly smooth foot soles – there are no creases yet.

If your baby is a girl, her clitoris will seem quite prominent. Neither this, nor her vaginal area, will yet have grown around them the protective folds of labia. If your

Ryan, born at 28 weeks

Why premature babies are thin

It is completely normal for premature babies to be thin, and the thinness is only temporary. They were born before they would have naturally started building up their layers of fat; in the womb this begins at about 32–34 weeks. A premature baby who is healthy will usually begin to put on a little fat from around 32 weeks.

However, coping with the outside world before they are ready makes huge demands upon premature babies' systems. They need to use all their calories and energy for surviving and developing, and have little left over to spend on getting fatter.

They are also under a great deal of stress, having to deal with things that they are not yet physically ready for – such as bright light, noise, touch, discomfort, pain or even breathing air. Just how much stress your baby may be under depends a great deal on how he is being looked after and protected, how well or unwell he is and how early he was born. But as he becomes stronger and more mature, he will be able to cope more easily.

When he no longer has to use all his energy just surviving, he will have some to spare for storing up in the form of fat padding and he will become chubbier.

baby is a boy, his testes will not have descended, and will still be tucked up inside his body. No nipples are visible on either girls or boys.

What your baby may be able to do

At this gestational age babies do not often have the energy to move much, but they may be quite active if they become agitated. Although his limbs are not strong, your baby may sometimes like to stretch, as he used to do in your womb, and may occasionally bring his hand up to his mouth to try and suck his thumb or fingers, clamp his fingers into a fist or splay them open, or turn his head. If he can open his eyes for a few moments he may be able to see simple black and white patterns. He can hear sound; and he can certainly feel pain: all premature babies, no matter how early they were born, can feel pain.

Your baby can communicate using facial expressions and body language: yawning, hiccuping, arching his back, splaying his fingers (see page 86). He will probably be able to recognize voices – especially his mother's, perhaps also his father's, and maybe his brothers' and sisters' voices too.

From around week 28–29 onwards, depending on how well or strong he is, your baby may be able to lick at breast-milk expressed from your nipples, as a first step towards breast-feeding, and he may begin to learn to cup-feed (see page 116).

What your baby may not yet be able to do

He cannot lie curled up in the fetal position unless he is supported gently to do so (see page 93) but lies with his arms and legs sprawled out sideways. This is because his limbs do not yet have any active muscle tone. (This will start developing at around 34–36 weeks.) He won't be able to lift his head, and he may not be able to cry. More importantly, there are three vital things he probably cannot do for himself. He can't breathe all the time without help. He can't keep himself warm. And he can't feed for himself. He will probably be able to suck, but premature babies of this age cannot co-ordinate their sucking, swallowing and breathing. This means he can't yet drink from your breast or a bottle without choking on the milk.

When your baby was inside you, he never had to worry about any of these things. Everything he needed you supplied, or did for him. He was warm in the shelter of your body. He did not need to breathe or eat because both food and oxygen came through the placenta and down through his lifeline, the umbilical cord. Now he is going to need some help for a while, until his systems are mature enough to take over.

For a description of the help your baby will be given, please see *What happens now?*, pages 22–81.

IF YOUR BABY IS BORN AT 29 TO 34 WEEKS

If your baby is born 11 to 6 weeks early, he will probably weigh between just over 1,000g and 2,500g (2–5½lb) and be about 30–35cm (12–14in) long.

How your baby may look

At 29 weeks he will not yet look like a smaller version of the traditional pink, chubby newborn. He will still have some growing, developing and, most of all, some weight-gaining to do. But a premature baby from 34 weeks upwards may well be starting to look much more like a newborn term baby.

However his head will not yet be in proportion with his body, and he will look thin. Some of his blood vessels may still show slightly through his skin; but these will become harder to see over the next few weeks, as he begins to build up a layer of fat. He will have soft downy hairs – called lanugo – on his face and body, especially his back. This developed naturally in the womb and will disappear over the next few weeks.

His small ears are floppy and do not yet spring back if they are folded down. This is because the cartilage which keeps ears in shape under pressure has not finished developing. The soles of his feet are relatively smooth, only having one or two creases on them. If your baby is a girl, her clitoris and inner labia will be fairly prominent and visible, because the outer folds of protective skin and soft tissue which form both labia have not yet finished growing. If your baby is a boy, you will see that his scrotum looks smoother than an older baby's. On both boys and girls, you can see the beginnings of nipples measuring

Wrinkle-free

Most medical books seem to say that premature babies have wrinkled skin. They haven't – unless they are born very dehydrated, which is not common these days.

The myth dates back 30 years or more to the time when if a baby was born prematurely he was usually very dehydrated too, and this out-of-date information has stayed in the textbooks.

Ellen, born just seconds ago, after 34 weeks in the womb

1–2mm across on their chests, though these are a fainter colour than a term baby's.

What your baby may be able to do

He will be able to move his arms, legs, and body – sometimes quite vigorously – and his head from side to side. He may be able to grasp your finger firmly. He could probably suck on a dummy if you gave him one and may be able to nuzzle at, and perhaps begin practice sucking on, his mother's nipple for comfort. If you express a few drops of milk and leave them on your nipple, your baby may be able to lick these off like a kitten – or even begin to try and breast-feed. Given the right support and help, he may be able to cup-feed from a special tiny, round-edged cup, licking and lapping at the milk (see page 116).

He may be able to turn his head towards the sound of your voice or another sound that draws his attention, and focus with interest on a face or picture about 25cm (10in) away (this is also the distance between his face and yours if you are holding him in your arms to feed him). He is likely to be able to recognize his parents' faces and/or voices – and perhaps his brothers' or sisters' too. He can feel pain, he can cry, and he can probably stay awake for short periods (beginning with a couple of minutes), alert and watchful, eyes wide open. He can communicate using facial expressions and body language and may be able to interact with you a little.

What your baby may not yet be able to do

He can't lie with his arms and legs curled close to his body in the fetal position, as you would expect a newborn baby to do, unless he is positioned in the right way and gently supported (see page 93). Instead, as he has so little muscle tone, your baby will lie with his arms and legs slightly akimbo, sprawled out to the sides. Nor can he yet hold his head up, if you pull him gently into a sitting position.

Although he may be able to suck strongly, he is unlikely to be able to breast- or bottle-feed. Until they are around 34 weeks, premature babies find it difficult to manage to co-ordinate sucking, swallowing and breathing regularly and in the right order. This is why trying to drink

How can a 3,400g (7½lb) baby be 'premature'?

True, this is the average weight of a baby who has been in the womb for 40 weeks. Yet it is not just your baby's actual weight which is important at this stage, but also how mature his body systems are. Each extra week in the womb gives all these systems – breathing, digestion, temperature control, vision – vital extra time to develop.

A 3,400g (7½lb), 35-week baby may be a good size but still need a little extra help in these areas, even if it is only for a short while.

The help your baby needs

Premature babies may need a lot of extra care. Much of this, especially if they are very premature or unwell, is specialized medical care, and the next chapter details the many ways in which the hospital can help.

But babies have great need of their parents too, and there is an enormous amount that loving mothers and fathers can do to help, nurture and protect even the most fragile or tiny premature baby; if you would like to find out some more about this, please see *What can we do?* on pages 82–127.

milk by mouth may make them choke, so they need to take most of their food by tube. Your baby will need extra help in keeping warm, and he will probably not be able to breathe without some help. Until they are around 36 weeks GA, premature babies' lungs do not produce enough surfactant – the substance that coats the inside of the lungs' airways and air sacs to help them stay open between breaths. Without enough surfactant, lungs collapse. This is why most premature babies will temporarily need some breathing support, ranging from a little extra oxygen to a ventilator (see pages 28–33).

IF YOUR BABY IS BORN AT 35 TO 37 WEEKS

If your baby was born 5 to 3 weeks early, he will probably weigh anything from 1,600–3,400g (3½–7½lb) and be about 38–45cm (15–18in) long.

How your baby may look

At this gestational age, a premature baby will often look little different from a term baby. He may still have some of the soft downy hair called lanugo, which formed naturally in the womb, on his body, and perhaps on his face too, but this will soon disappear. He will probably be thinner than you would expect a term newborn baby to be. This is because the last few weeks in the womb is spent putting on weight (see page 16).

His fingernails and toenails may not quite touch the ends of their digits. If your baby is a girl, her outer labia may not completely cover her inner labia, vaginal opening and clitoris yet. If he is a boy, both his testes may not have dropped into place. Sometimes only one will have done so, or either one or both testes will sometimes move back up into his body again. When this happens it is called having retractable testes.

What your baby may be able to do

If your baby is well and stable, he may now be beginning to cope with and do many more of the things that you might notice a newborn term baby doing. At around 37 weeks, his hands might be strong enough to hold tight to your fingers, as you slowly and gently pull him up. He may try to hold his head steady, and if you are holding him in a sitting position, he may try to bring his head up off his chest and hold it there for several seconds. Younger premature babies' movements tend to be weak and jerky, but your baby may now be able to move his arms and legs fairly strongly and smoothly and to bring his hands up to his mouth, sucking his fingers.

He will probably see almost as well as a term baby and enjoy looking at faces and patterns. He may try to follow your face with his eyes or turn his head to follow the sound of your voice, and crane to look up at you as you hold him close to your chest. He will probably recognize his mother's and father's voices, and perhaps any older brothers' or sisters' voices too. He may coo, or try to.

What your baby may not yet be able to do
If your baby is well, there may be little that a newborn term baby can do that he can't. However, even if he is able to breast-feed, bottle-feed or feed from a cup (see page 116) he may also need some temporary extra help in the form of tube-feeding. He may need help with breathing (perhaps just a little extra oxygen from time to time) and he will probably need extra heating to keep warm.

THE DEVELOPMENT OF THE BRAIN
There is a huge difference between what a 26- or 27-week GA premature baby can do and cope with, and what (if he is well and being cared for properly) he will be able to manage just 6 short weeks later at 32–33 weeks. This is partly because the brain of a 26-week baby is very different from a 33-week baby's. The brain's surface, and therefore its capacity, develops very fast between weeks 24 and 40.

Another important thing which happens in the 24–40 week period and helps a baby's brain to work more efficiently is that the system of ultra-fine 'electrical wiring' that connects the brain and nerve cells together starts developing insulation. This process is called myelination. The signals passing from one brain cell to another are tiny electric charges and if they are to travel efficiently their pathways need to be insulated so they do not 'leak'. Myelin is the substance that develops to insulate the nerve fibres.

The surface of the brain
A 24-week-old premature baby's brain is smooth-surfaced, almost like a tennis ball. A 40-week-old term baby's looks more like a huge walnut. This is because from 24 weeks' gestation onwards, the brain's surface has been folding itself into an intricate mass of ridges. And it is those ridges that are vital for learning and intelligence.

The brain's surface is the business part of the brain, the intelligent part. The surface cells are connected with the brain centre, then the spine and body, by fibres which make up the bulk of the brain itself. The bigger a brain's surface area is, the more of those neurological connections it can make and so the more information it can process.

The folding, wrinkling process which goes on between 24 and 40 weeks is important because it increases a baby's brain's surface area enormously without taking up more room inside the skull. The end result is that the brain becomes far more powerful and efficient, so its owner can cope with more, do more and learn more.

What happens now?

Names and abbreviations

★ Neonatal care is the specialist care of newborn (including premature) babies

★ *SCBU: Special Care Baby Unit*, which provides care for babies who need more than the usual level of neonatal care

★ *Intensive care* involves a major degree of advanced technological support and top-level staff expertise

★ *NICU: Neonatal Intensive Care Unit*, which provides the most sophisticated level of care for babies, is to be found at major hospitals and centres of excellence

Your baby may now be in the unfamiliar world of the Special Care Baby Unit and this chapter will try to introduce and explain the procedures and therapies she may experience and the machines, tubes and equipment surrounding her. It also looks at the possible reasons why your baby may need medical treatment – both minor medical problems that premature babies may have, and more serious medical conditions.

This chapter also looks at some of the many things that you, as your baby's mother and father, can do to help her, but for more detailed information, please see the chapter *What can we do?* on pages 82–127. Your love, care, watchfulness and protection are every bit as important to your baby's recovery as the skill of professional medical staff and the complex technology of the unit.

WHAT ARE ALL THOSE TUBES?

The first things that may strike you when you go into a neonatal unit are the heat, the bright lights and the number of machines that are in constant use. The initial impression for parents and visitors can be of a science fiction world, whose complex equipment dwarfs the small babies being cared for there.

It can be both frightening and upsetting to see your baby lying in an incubator, attached to tubes and wires, watched over by monitors that constantly flash and bleep. Yet most parents say that they found that the more they knew about what the equipment was all for and how the different pieces of it were helping their baby, the less intimidating it became. If there is anything you are not sure about, the neonatal staff will be willing and happy to help you. Don't worry if you find you need to ask the same questions again and again. The nurses will expect this, and they will understand. They recognize that when someone is worried, tired and stressed (and you may be feeling all three) it can be very difficult to remember even very basic information clearly the first time around. If you do not quite understand what a certain piece of equipment does, then many other parents before you – and many who will be at the unit after you – didn't or won't either. And as your baby's parents, if you need to know something, however small, then it is important.

GENERAL EQUIPMENT IN THE SPECIAL CARE BABY UNIT

A premature baby may be born needing help with three very important and basic things: keeping warm, breathing and feeding. The equipment you see on a neonatal unit will either be helping your baby do any, or all, of these, or monitoring her to see how she is managing, and checking whether she needs any additional support.

What follows is a general guide to the type of equipment you may see used to help your baby. Specific resources and procedures vary from hospital to hospital.

Incubator

An incubator is basically a transparent plastic box on wheels. Its job is to keep your baby warm. Underneath it there is usually a cupboard for her things, such as nappies and any clothing. There are two main types of incubator:

Closed incubators have a lid, porthole windows and are double glazed to keep in heat. A closed or lidded incubator also controls the amount of humidity (water) in the air surrounding your baby. This is important, as the hot, dry air of the neonatal unit can dry out their vulnerable skin. Small or sick premature babies may lose a good deal of water through their skins because they cannot control their own body temperature.

Open incubators have no lid or portholes. However they do have an overhead heating unit, and sometimes a specially heated mattress as well.

As your baby progresses and finds it easier to control her own body temperature, she will be able to move to an open Perspex cot which has no heater.

Vital signs monitors

Vital signs is the term used for the markers that show how well your baby's major body systems are working.

To check all or any of these vital signs, your baby may be attached to a monitoring system, via small sensor pads with lead wires which are stuck to her chest. Several

'We used to write everything down in a book and keep that in the cupboard under her incubator so we could look it up again if we forgot what a tube or machine did. We were always forgetting at first, it seems such a lot to take in. Later, it got so that we were explaining it all to visitors like a pair of nurses...'

Marianne, mother of Sharina, who was born at 33 weeks

Vital signs include your baby's

* Breathing rate
* Heart rate (pulse)
* Blood pressure
* Temperature
* Blood gasses. This means the amounts of oxygen and carbon dioxide in your baby's bloodstream and also how acidic or alkaline her blood is.

separate monitors can now be combined into a single machine that shows information for some, or all, of the vital signs on a TV-style screen. Which vital signs they will be monitoring depends on how well or unwell your baby is at the moment.

A **cardiorespiratory monitor** is a vital signs monitor that measures heart rate and breathing rate. An alarm goes off if either gets too far above or below the normal level.

A **pulse oximeter**, sometimes also called a **saturation monitor**, measures the amount of oxygen in a baby's blood using an infra-red light sensor, which is usually attached to the baby's hand or foot. Monitoring oxygen is vital when a premature baby is sick. Too little or too much can be harmful, and may cause long-term health problems.

There are two main types of **blood pressure monitor**. Your baby's blood pressure can be measured either by wrapping a cuff (a mini version of the type used for adults) around her upper arm or by using a device attached to a line going into an artery. In either case the results are fed into a machine that automatically measures and then displays the pressure reading.

Ambient oxygen analyser

This is a small device placed inside the incubator. It checks the amount of oxygen in the surrounding air.

IV line

IV stands for *intravenous* – the word comes from the Latin for inside a vein. An IV line is a fine tube threaded into one of your baby's main veins. It may be in her arm, leg, scalp or umbilical cord. If she is very unwell or very premature, she can be fed through this tube. She can also be given extra fluids, extra nutrients or medications down her IV line. These are gently pumped through by a device called a **syringe driver**.

Naso-gastric (NG) tube; oro-gastric (OG) tube; transpyloric tube

These are fine, flexible, plastic feeding tubes. A naso-gastric tube is threaded through the baby's nose, an oro-gastric through her mouth, down her throat and into her

A Vital signs monitor
B Electronic thermometer
C Pumps which control the amount of fluid being fed through a drip to the baby

Alarming alarms

The sound of monitor alarms ringing is the backing track of every SCBU. It never seems to stop (especially in the intensive care room) and it can be stressful for babies, staff and parents alike. Yet you may have seen that the nurses do not always seem to react.

In nearly every case this is not because they haven't noticed; they almost certainly have, but they know from experience that this is not an alarm that needs a medical response – this time.

This gets easier to cope with as you get to know and trust your baby's regular nurses and they get to know you and your baby. However, at first it can be very worrying and frustrating – and some parents remember it made them downright angry.

If you are worried, it may help to try and talk to the staff about your concerns and they should be able to explain how and when they think a medical response is appropriate – and when not to worry.

stomach. A transpyloric tube goes directly to the baby's small intestine.

Umbilical catheter sensors

These fine plastic tubes are passed through an artery or vein in the baby's tummy button (umbilicus). They can be used for giving her fluids, nutrients and medications, or for taking blood samples. Some SCBUs also attach to these lines special machines that can measure your baby's blood pressure and/or the level of oxygen in her bloodstream.

Phototherapy unit

This is a lamp unit that shines bright light – not ultra violet light – on to a baby's naked skin. It is used to help treat jaundice, usually successfully (see page 45).

Biliblanket

This is a special mat, made up of soft fibre-optic tubes that give out bright light, which the baby lies on. Biliblankets are used as another way of giving a jaundiced baby phototherapy treatment.

Apnoea alarm

If a baby stops breathing for more than 10–20 seconds, she is having an apnoea attack (see page 34). This is a common problem for premature babies, though most have stopped having these attacks before they leave hospital.

In the meantime, your baby may need either to wear an apnoea alarm around her tummy, or to lie on a special flat alarm pad placed underneath her mattress. The alarm will sound if she stops breathing for a certain (brief) period of time. Very occasionally, a baby may go home with one of these alarms (see page 172).

SPECIAL EQUIPMENT TO HELP WITH BREATHING

Many premature babies have problems with their lungs, and need some extra help with their breathing. Some may only need a little help for a few days. Others may need hi-tech support from a ventilator for many weeks, even, occasionally, months.

Extra oxygen, headboxes and oxygen masks

This equipment is used for babies who can breathe without help but need some extra oxygen. Air with extra oxygen added to it can be delivered straight into a covered incubator. It may also be piped into a special clear Perspex box called a **headbox** which rests over the baby's head, or delivered via an **oxygen mask**. Both the boxes and the masks can be used in an open incubator.

Nasal cannula

This is a way of giving a baby extra oxygen through the nose, using two tiny tubes (one in each nostril). These are attached to slim, flexible plastic piping that goes back across each cheek, behind the baby's ears and then along to the source of oxygen.

Archie is being fed through a naso-gastric tube, and a nasal cannula is helping him to breathe.

Oxygen analyser

Whenever a baby needs extra oxygen, the level is always measured very carefully by an analyser. This is usually a small plastic sensor placed near the baby's face or somewhere along the oxygen route.

Humidifier

If your baby needs long-term oxygen therapy, the air and oxygen mixture is often passed through a humidifier first. This moistens and warms the gasses: something that a term baby's nose does naturally.

CPAP

This stands for *continuous positive airway pressure*. It usually involves a mixture of air and extra oxygen being blown, through two small tubes placed in the baby's nostrils, into her nose and down into her lungs to help keep the air sacs open after each breath. It keeps them slightly inflated – as they are in an adult or a term baby – even after exhaling, to ensure that they do not collapse inwards, and prevents the inner surfaces sticking together. The result is that the baby does not have to make such an effort to draw each breath. CPAP can also be given via an endotracheal tube (see below).

Ventilator

This is a machine that either helps a baby to breathe or, if necessary, can take over the process completely. A mixture of air and extra oxygen is gently blown or pushed down a pipe called an **endotracheal tube (ET)**. The tube leads from her mouth, down her throat and into her lungs. Some babies may need ventilator support for just a day or two, others may need it for many weeks or even months.

There are several different sorts of ventilator. A large regional neonatal unit may offer them all, though a small SCBU may only have one or two. The type of ventilator a baby will have depends on the sort of problems she is experiencing. If she needs a special ventilator which the unit does not have, she may well be transferred to a bigger unit that does. There are two main types of ventilator:

A **positive pressure ventilator** pushes a mixture of air and extra oxygen under carefully controlled pressure

Being attached to a naso-gastric tube doesn't stop Ellen enjoying a cuddle. (She's doing her best to pull the tube out, though.)

through a soft ET. This air flows down into the baby's lungs, and helps them to expand normally as she breathes in. Breathing out again follows naturally when the machine stops puffing the air, allowing the baby's chest to fall again. The ventilator puffs down 20–40 'breaths' a minute, on average. A baby will stay on the ventilator until her lungs are mature enough to cope alone, or have healed from whatever damage they have suffered. The weaning-off-the-ventilator process is careful and gradual.

Some positive pressure ventilators are highly sophisticated. For babies who cannot breathe without help at all, they will do all the necessary work. Other babies can cope with taking at least some breaths themselves, and the machine can allow them to do this in between ventilator breaths. There are also some types of positive pressure ventilator which babies can trigger themselves.

CPAP helps George to breathe. He is being fed through an oro-gastric tube, and his vital signs are constantly monitored via the sensor pads stuck to his chest.

These machines wait for a baby to begin to take a breath herself, then gently blow in some extra air mixture at the same time to give a helping hand.

An **oscillatory ventilator** or **high-frequency ventilator** still uses an ET to deliver the air mixture into the baby's lungs. But it delivers smaller puffs of air and extra oxygen at a much faster rate: instead of being blown down, the gas is 'vibrated' down. A baby supported by this type of machine does not look as if she is breathing, as such, at all. Her chest doesn't rise and fall, but shakes with vibrations. This type of ventilator is much gentler on the lungs.

ORDINARY MEDICAL PROBLEMS

Because your baby has been born ahead of her time, her body is not yet ready to adapt to life outside the shelter of your womb and she may have some difficulties at first. Here are some of the most common problems a premature baby may need to deal with, together with information about all the things that both the SCBU and you, as your baby's parents, can do to help your child.

Please don't read this section straight through from start to finish. It is only about the *possible* health problems your baby may face -- it is not a list of all the illnesses she will definitely have. Many are either completely normal things for premature babies to experience temporarily, or they are common conditions which can be treated easily and effectively. Try to treat this part of the book as a reference section to dip into when you want to know something about a specific problem. It is far more likely that your baby will only develop, say, two or three of the difficulties mentioned in this section, and then only for a short time. Most of these will either sort themselves out as your child's system matures, or they can be treated by the SCBU staff without any lasting ill effects at all.

Many of the most common health problems for a premature baby, such as difficulty keeping warm, apnoea and cyanosis, happen because her nervous system has not yet finished maturing, so it cannot yet keep many of the body functions stable and even. The more premature a

Serious problems

The more premature a baby is, the more difficulties she may experience and the more serious these may be; the less premature she is, the fewer and less serious the difficulties are likely to be.

For less usual but more severe problems, please see the section starting on page 57.

'Every time she stopped breathing for even a few seconds, it was like my own heart stopped. We tried to be cool about it, like some of the other parents who would just sigh, and rub their baby's feet to get things going again. But we just never could get quite used to it.'

Steven, father of Chloe, born at 34 weeks

baby is, the more of a problem she will have with this, though babies can mature surprisingly fast if they are basically well, and properly cared for. There are enormous differences between what a 28-week premature baby can handle and what a 34-weeker can manage.

BREATHING PAUSES (APNOEA)

Premature babies often stop breathing for a few moments. As a matter of fact, so do many newborn term babies. If the pauses only last from 5–10 seconds before they re-start by themselves, the condition is called periodic breathing. This periodic breathing is a harmless and perfectly normal thing for a new baby to do, and because it doesn't cause a baby any problems it doesn't need any treatment. However, if your baby's breathing pauses are longer, say nearer 10–20 seconds long, this is known as apnoea. These breathing pauses may cause her heartbeat to slow (this is called bradycardia, see page 36) and her skin to become pale, mottled or bluish. Afro-Caribbean babies tend to show they are short of oxygen by having darker lips, a darker area around their noses and a darker colour than usual on their tongues.

Most premature babies have apnoea. Some studies have found that they spend as much as 12 per cent of their breathing time pausing. The more premature your baby is, the more likely she is to have apnoea, and the more mature a baby is at birth, the less likely. Apnoea is usually caused by the immaturity of your baby's nervous system and lungs and airways; though in some cases there may be something blocking her breathing tube – for instance, her tongue may relax back into her throat while she is asleep because it does not yet have enough muscle tone to keep itself in its proper position.

Apnoea tends to start, if it is going to, within a day or two of a premature baby's being born. It only lasts until her breathing and central nervous systems mature, which may take anything from a few days to several weeks. If your baby is on a ventilator, this hides signs of apnoea, which may then appear when she begins breathing on her own.

However frequently your baby pauses for breath, you can expect a big improvement when she reaches 31–33 weeks (gestational age).

What staff may do to help

Often no one will need to do anything, as your baby will usually start breathing again on her own. If she doesn't breathe within 20 seconds or so, a nurse will help her to start breathing again by gently rubbing or stroking her side or foot. If this doesn't work, staff will try giving extra oxygen. They may do so by gently blowing a stream of oxygen near your baby's face; or by 'bagging' – carefully pumping extra oxygen into your baby's lungs using a small oxygen bag, plus a mask.

If a premature baby has frequent apnoea spells, staff will monitor her carefully so that they can act fast if any trouble develops, or she may have extra help with her breathing for a while.

Checking and helping your baby's breathing

The medical staff may attach her to a pulse oximeter (see page 26) that tracks the amount of oxygen in her blood. Alternatively – or perhaps as well – she may be connected to a cardiorespiratory monitor (see page 26) to keep a check on her heartbeat and breathing rate. Both machines have alarms that go off if your baby's oxygen levels, heartbeat or breathing rate drop even slightly below a certain level. Or she may just be attached to an apnoea alarm (see page 28).

Your baby could also be given some continuous help for a while. This may be in the form of nasal CPAP (see page 30) or medicines, such as theophylline or caffeine, to stimulate the central nervous system.

What parents can do

Although it can be really alarming to see your baby's breathing pause, try not to panic. It's completely natural to react strongly if you see your baby stop breathing for even a few seconds – those few seconds can seem like a very long time – but premature babies can take far longer breathing pauses than adults can without any apparent ill effects. If possible, try not to focus only on the breathing pauses or, in isolation, on the readings on any monitor she may be connected to. Instead, look at your baby closely to see how well or comfortable she seems and how healthy

Medicine-watch

If your baby is being given theophylline or caffeine, keep an eye on her behaviour. Staff will be monitoring her too, by maintaining a careful record of the levels of theophylline in her bloodstream (though they tend not to check caffeine levels).

Both types of drug are very useful for apnoea, and caffeine is useful for bradycardia, but their side-effects can include restlessness and irritability, and they may occasionally make a premature baby vomit or send her heart rate up.

If any of these reactions occur, ask your baby's carers whether perhaps another approach that doesn't have these side-effects could be used for a while instead.

If a premature baby is on medication that is making her unsettled, this will affect her rest and sleep, which are vital to her growth and recovery.

her colour is, because these are things that are just as important.

If the breathing pauses are too long, you need not feel you have to stand by and do nothing. Try rubbing your baby's feet gently but firmly. This will usually stimulate her to begin breathing normally again. If it does not work within 20 seconds, call a nurse to help you.

Outlook

The likely outcome for your baby is excellent. Premature babies grow out of apnoea as their breathing systems mature. Many parents worry that there might be a link between apnoea and the likelihood of cot death (see page 171). However, the most recent UK study about this (1996) suggests that although premature babies are more vulnerable to cot death than babies born at term, this is because they are more likely to have a range of health problems – not because they have experienced and then grown out of apnoea spells.

SLOWING HEARTBEAT (BRADYCARDIA)

The hearts of most premature babies beat roughly 120 to 160 times a minute (this is about twice as fast as yours). If your baby's heartbeat slows down to less than 100 beats a minute, this is known as bradycardia. This temporary slowing of the heart is most usually caused by an apnoea spell but, occasionally, bradycardia may be the effect of a heart problem.

What staff may do to help

The staff's response to bradycardia will generally be similar to their treatment of apnoea (see page 35). They will rub your baby's foot gently but firmly, and if that doesn't have the desired effect, they may give her some extra oxygen. They may also keep a check on her by attaching her to a cardiorespiratory monitor (see page 26), and if they think some continuous help is necessary they may give her caffeine medication. However, in many instances they may do nothing, except watch the baby carefully. The slowing might not be too far from the normal range and she may recover without any help.

What parents can do

Rub your baby's foot gently but firmly. If this doesn't seem to help, or if you are worried about her because she seems distressed or doesn't look well, ask a nurse to come over to check on her.

Outlook

The likely outcome for your baby is excellent. So long as the bradycardia spells are not caused by a heart problem, she will grow out of them as her nervous system and breathing mechanisms mature.

TEMPORARILY BLUISH SKIN (CYANOSIS)

Babies' skin often has this blue tinge in the first few hours after they have been born, especially if they are cold. No

Storm now breathes on her own, but extra oxygen can be piped into her headbox whenever she needs it.

matter how warm delivery rooms may be they are up to 11C (20°F) colder than it was inside you.

If your baby has slightly bluish fingers and toes, this is likely to be what doctors call **peripheral cyanosis**, which is caused by the immaturity of her circulation control system. This can lead to congestion (sluggish circulation), but is not usually a problem.

However, if your baby has a bluish colour around her mouth, bluish tongue, lips or an all-over bluish-pink or 'dusky' skin tone, she may well have the more serious **central cyanosis**. On darker-skinned or Afro-Caribbean babies the bluish tinge is not so easy to see, though experienced neonatal staff can spot it. Often a colour change can be seen inside a darker-skinned baby's mouth or on her tongue, or a paler area around her nose and mouth.

Central cyanosis needs to be dealt with urgently because it means that your baby is not getting enough oxygen. There can be many reasons for this, including the possibilities that: her heart may not be pumping oxygen-rich blood round her body fast or effectively enough; she may not be breathing effectively; she may have an infection; or she may be cold.

What staff may do to help

If apnoea seems to be the cause of the trouble, they will rub your baby's feet gently to re-stimulate her breathing. If the breathing problems are more serious, they may give her some extra oxygen or further assist her breathing. If she is too cold, they will give her extra warmth and make sure she keeps warm.

What parents can do

Rub your baby's feet gently if she is having an apnoea spell, and see if she is warm enough by feeling the back of her neck or her body; it is not a good idea to check her body temperature by feeling her hands and feet – these may give a wrong impression because, as her circulation is not mature yet, they are very often chillier than the rest of her body. If you are still worried, ask a nurse to come and check your baby.

Outlook

Unless the cyanosis is due to a serious health problem – for example an abnormality in the way your baby's heart has developed or a lung condition such as BPD (see page 60) – she will grow out of it naturally as her breathing system and heart mature.

FRAGILE SKIN

A premature baby's skin is very delicate. It has a far thinner fatty bottom layer than a term baby's, and the top layer is thin and fragile, so it doesn't protect the middle growing layer well and it's not so securely attached. Your baby's skin will be thinner than a term baby's; it will tend to be dry, to absorb anything put on it too readily and to be easily damaged – even the gentle removal of a sticking plaster can cause a minor wound. Therefore it can easily get infected. The earlier a baby is born, the more delicate her skin will be.

What staff may do to help

There are many things the staff can do to minimize damage to your baby's fragile skin. They may use special medical tape for securing things like IV lines and dressings and can put soft barriers between your baby's skin and the sticky part of the tape. For example, dabbing any sticky tape that is going to be laid against her skin lightly against cotton wool coats the tape in a light protective fluff; this makes it less likely to remove any delicate skin when the tape is taken off again. When sticky tape needs to be taken off, the nurses can use warm water or a substance called Zoff to loosen it first, before pulling it away gently. Your baby's carers will use warm water only – no soaps – for washing her, and not put creams, lotions or other substances on her skin unless absolutely necessary, because they can be absorbed too easily.

Because the air in the SCBU is so hot and dry, it takes vital moisture from your baby's skin. The drier the skin is, the more likely it is to tear or crack, so staff may add water vapour to the baby's environment in the incubator to keep the air around her more humid. They will always try to touch your baby as gently as possible and may wrap her in

Skin

Skin is actually made up of three layers.

1 **Epidermis**: the protective top layer

2 **Dermis**: the middle or growing layer

3 **Subcutaneous tissue**: the fatty bottom layer which helps keep out the cold.

Together the layers act as a barrier against the outside world.

Flaky skin

Your baby's skin is likely to go through a quite normal dry and flaky stage as it matures: try to resist the powerful temptation to put on creams to moisten it – it won't help in the long run. If you are worried that your baby is not comfortable, talk to a senior member of staff to see what they can suggest.

a soft material called paraffin gauze for extra protection. Cling film is also used to protect fragile premature skin and keep its moisture in.

What parents can do

Try to make sure that anyone who touches and handles your baby does so very gently. Check that her nurses do use some sort of effective barrier between her skin and any sticky medical tape securing IV lines. If they are not doing this, and especially if you notice a sore place on your baby's skin where tape has removed a small area of it, talk about it to a senior member of staff whom you like and trust, such as one of the nursing sisters or the neonatologist in charge of the unit.

Outlook

Your baby's skin may be immature but it is growing up fast. Within a few weeks the top layer will be almost as securely attached and strong as any newborn term baby's, and it will be less dry and flaky.

LOSING WEIGHT / NOT GAINING WEIGHT

It's normal for babies to lose weight just after they are born, whether they have spent their full quota of 38–41 weeks in your womb, or arrived early. There are usually two (generally harmless) reasons for this. First, your baby is getting rid of the extra water and salt in her system that she doesn't need any more; she had a lot of both when she was still in your womb. Secondly, term and later-born, more mature premature babies being breast-fed will for the first few days be receiving colostrum, or pre-milk. This marvellous fluid is rich in minerals, vitamins and antibodies to fight infection, but not high in the calories that help a baby put on weight.

Even when your baby begins to gain weight, she may not put it on steadily at first. Premature babies need more calories because everything is more of an effort for them, and they may be taking in less food than they need. If they are distressed or uncomfortable, they may spend energy (calories) trying to cope with this, or moving frantically. Very premature babies have a higher metabolic rate too,

Weight loss

The smaller or more premature babies are when they are born, or the more unwell they are, the more weight they will lose at first. Full-term babies lose 5–10 per cent of their weight just after they are born, but premature babies lose nearer to 10–15 per cent.

and this is another reason why they may need more food than they are able to take in.

Premature babies have tiny stomachs and can only take a little nourishment at a time. However, provided they are well, their stomachs can usually hold enough food for their needs if they are fed at least every two to four hours. (Some babies may need to be fed a tiny amount continuously via a drip or a tube.) Problems arise if something, say repeated vomiting, is stopping your baby from taking in and retaining the food she needs. If she has a gut problem, this will also prevent her from absorbing enough from the milk she has taken in.

What the staff may do to help

The nursing staff will set up a careful feeding regime and measure your baby's weight and growth regularly – daily if she is unstable or unwell, or every few days if she seems to be growing steadily. They will make very sure she is getting enough fluids. Just how much your baby needs is calculated exactly, even down to the number of drops needed per minute for some very small babies.

Your baby is likely to be losing water through her thin, fragile skin, so staff will try to make up for this by adding extra humidity (moisture) to her cot. They will also make sure she stays warm, so that she does not waste calories trying to generate her own central heating. If that vital energy has to be spent on keeping warm it cannot be used for growing. The staff should generally also be trying to keep your baby calm and comfortable. Stress and restlessness also use up the calories your baby needs to spend on growing.

What parents can do

If you spend a lot of time watching your baby carefully you will be in the best position to judge whether she is comfortable. Anything you can do that reassures her, comforts her or helps keep her calm can be really valuable: the more comfortable your baby is, the more calories she can save for growing and putting on weight. There are many things that you, as your baby's parents, can do to help make your child calmer and more comfortable, even

'Every day we'd ask: "Has she gained?" and would worry if she hadn't, or even worse, had lost weight. A good day for us was her putting weight on, a bad day was when she lost some …'

Martine and John, mother and father of Zoe, who was born at 29 weeks

Premature babies get cold very easily for three main reasons.

1 They are born before they have laid down much fat under their skin, so do not have much natural heat insulation.

2 When older babies and adults are cold they generate their own extra heat by shivering. Newborn babies cannot shiver, and for emergency heat supplies they burn up a special sort of fat, called brown fat, instead. Premature babies have very little of that, and none at all if they are less than 30 weeks old.

3 The bigger a body's surface area is relative to its weight, the faster heat is lost from it and the more easily it gets cold. All babies have a much bigger surface area relative to their weight than adults and the ratio for premature babies is even higher than for term babies, so they lose heat fastest.

A nurse takes Nina's temperature, using an electronic thermometer. The baby's hat is a vital piece of equipment, preventing her from losing heat through her head.

if she is very unwell; there are some ideas and suggestions in the next chapter, *What can we do?*

Try not to be discouraged if your baby loses weight for a couple of days, even if she had been putting it on steadily before. This is normal. Every baby is unique, and they all have their own special patterns for putting weight on – maybe gaining for a few days, staying still for a couple, then losing weight again for a couple. You can get a clearer idea of how your baby is doing if you average out her weight gain over a week. It also a good idea to take a long look at the baby herself: that will tell you more than just a weight chart every time. How does she seem to you? Is her colour OK, does she seem fairly peaceful and comfortable? This can mean more than any temporary fall in weight.

Outlook

Your baby will grow bigger and stronger steadily as her body systems become more mature, though this may happen more slowly if she has been very unwell or was especially fragile to begin with.

KEEPING WARM

All premature babies need some extra help with keeping warm. But of all the things they need, this is the one that SCBUs can deal with most easily. Neonatal care units are very warm places anyway (which parents and staff know to their cost, as they are often uncomfortably hot for adults).

Unit staff will also use everything from incubators, overhead cot warmers and pre-warmed oxygen to blankets, baby bonnets and bubble wrap to help make sure your baby does not become chilly. Even so, both you and they need to keep a constant look-out for signs that your baby is cold (see page 162). Being cold can make a baby ill, because it may cause breathing problems, low blood sugar levels and weight loss.

Also, when premature babies get cold they have to use up some of the energy they get from food to make heat – and this is energy they needed to spend on growing. Most early-born babies have their work cut out to take in just

One very good way to keep your baby warm is by kangaroo care (see page 102). This is skin-to-skin contact with your baby, with her snuggled up on your chest or between your breasts, down inside your shirt. Your own body heat is a natural means of keeping a baby, especially a premature baby, warm and it can be a lovely way for both parents to soothe and feel close to their baby.

enough food to grow, so wasting energy on keeping warm slows down their growth and weight gain.

What staff may do to help

Everyday precautions against your baby's getting cold include warming up everything before it's used on, or for, the baby: hands, incubator, blankets, sheets, clothing, mattress, washing water, drying towels, incubator or crib – even warming up any extra oxygen the baby is being given so it doesn't arrive in a chilly stream. Staff may put a warmed blanket on any cold surfaces your baby is placed on, such as weighing scales or X-ray plates, even if it's only for a moment. They should protect her from draughts, keeping her cot away from doors in constant use, from windows and from potentially chilly outside walls.

Staff will monitor your baby's temperature regularly and if there is a problem, they will use incubators, heated mattresses and overhead warmers, sometimes putting side-guards on the warming unit or stretching plastic wrap over the sides and end of it and over your baby too. They may wrap your baby in clean bubble wrap, and will probably give her a soft cotton bonnet to wear all the time, as everyone, babies and adults alike, loses a lot of heat via the head. And they will probably not wash your baby very much because even when using warm water and a warm towel, some water will still evaporate off your baby's skin as she is being dried and this cools her body down fast.

What parents can do

See if your baby's nurses are taking the precautions outlined above – if they are not, ask if you can talk to them about the ways they can help keep a baby warm and which they might recommend for your child. When you hold your baby in your arms or on your lap, make sure she has a hat or baby bonnet on, and use a soft blanket to wrap around her.

If her temperature tends to fall easily at the moment, try to resist the understandable urge to wash her. It's very natural for parents to want to wash their child: this is part of the usual baby care mothers and fathers instinctively do for a newborn, and the wish to do so can be very strong.

You may feel you'd especially like to wash your baby or have the nurses do so if she has little flakes of matter on her skin, such as dried blood or the remains of the soft waxy substance called vernix which covered her skin when she was in your womb. Yet these will not cause an infection or hurt her in any way and in the interests of keeping your baby warm it may be best to leave washing for a while. Talk to the nurses about this if it is bothering you – perhaps just her face could be dabbed gently?

Outlook

As your baby grows stronger and bigger, she will be able to keep herself warm more easily.

JAUNDICE

Jaundice shows itself as a yellowish tinge to your baby's skin and/or gums and to the whites of the eyes. In darker-skinned or Afro-Caribbean babies, yellowing of the whites of the eyes is often the only visible sign (Caucasian babies may look as if they have a slight suntan). The yellow tinge is caused by a pigment called bilirubin, which is produced when old red blood cells are broken down. If the liver cannot remove bilirubin quickly enough, it builds up in the blood and gets deposited in the fatty layer just below the skin, showing through as a yellowish colour.

Jaundice itself is not a disease (although it can sometimes be a sign of some condition such as an under-performing liver) and it is very common in all newborn babies, full-term and premature alike. This is because all babies are born with extra red blood cells they no longer need outside the womb and, perhaps more importantly, it usually takes three to four days for even a newborn term baby's liver to start working efficiently enough to remove bilirubin from the blood. It is normal for premature babies' livers to take five to ten days to remove this yellow material, but it can take far longer. The more prematurely they were born, the longer it may take.

Generally harmless and straightforward to treat, jaundice is still a condition that no one can afford to ignore as it can sometimes be a sign that the liver is not working

Up to eight out of every ten premature babies develop what doctors and nurses call physiological (or 'newborn') jaundice – but so do up to six in every ten term babies.

properly. If it becomes severe, it can cause further problems, including possible brain damage. Even at its mildest jaundice may make your baby drowsy, slow to feed and listless, and since premature babies tend not to have much energy or feed very easily at first, this can make things worse.

What staff may do to help

Physiological or 'newborn' jaundice often clears spontaneously after a few days, but in any case staff will keep a close watch on your baby's bilirubin levels using simple blood tests. If they think she needs treatment to clear the jaundice, they will use phototherapy.

Phototherapy (treatment with bright lights) works by making the bilirubin molecules change their shape, into one that is easier for the body to get rid of. Your baby will

An orange headbox guards the baby's eyes from the bright lights being used to treat his jaundice, and the cloth draped over the top dims the light further. Air is being fed into his lungs through an endotracheal tube, while a covering of bubble wrap – and the essential bonnet – help to keep him warm.

lie in her cot, naked but for eye shields, under warm, bright lights which are left on 24 hours a day – in effect 'sun-bathing' her jaundice away. Sometimes a light fibre-optic blanket called a Biliblanket (see page 28) is used instead. Instead of a mask-style covering, she may have a space-age-looking orange Perspex shield covering her entire head to protect her eyes; with this she is free to look about, and can interact more with you instead of being effectively blindfolded.

While she is having phototherapy treatment, your baby may develop a light rash, but this will vanish after treatment stops. She may also be sleepier than she usually is and have either runnier bowel movements than normal or none at all. It is important that the staff give her extra fluids because, like sun-bathing, phototherapy can be dehydrating. Premature babies can lose nearly twice as much fluid as usual when they are having light treatment, so this is really important.

Phototherapy works so well that it is usually the only treatment a baby will need. However, if your baby is too severely jaundiced for phototherapy to be effective she may be given a blood transfusion. This takes one to two hours and will be carried out by a doctor who will not even need to move your baby from her cot. Sometimes a baby will need several exchange transfusions, spaced over a couple of weeks.

If the jaundice carries on for a long time, the doctors will check out possible causes including metabolic problems, thyroid disease, blockages in the baby's bile ducts or liver infection. Depending on the problem, treatment may be medication (metabolic and thyroid problems), surgery (blockages) or antibiotics (infections).

What parents can do

It is very helpful if you can be there to calm your baby when she has her regular heel prick blood tests that check her bilirubin levels. If they are not already doing so, ask the medical staff if they can use any of the methods outlined on the right to minimize the pain. Babies do not like blood tests and can sometimes get quite upset.

Blood tests – minimizing the pain

If the nurses warm your baby's foot in their hands (or if you do this for your baby yourself) before trying to take a blood sample, this can make it easier to take the sample, and her foot will be less likely to need uncomfortable squeezing.

Some units use local anaesthetic creams – either lignocaine or amethocaine – put on the skin up to half an hour before the prick to help deaden the area. Most specialists will not use the better-known EMLA cream (which can be given to term babies and toddlers or older children), as it gets absorbed too readily into a premature baby's fragile skin.

Premature babies find it especially hard to calm themselves down again after becoming distressed but if you are there to comfort and soothe your baby she will settle down again far more quickly.

You can still take your baby out from under the lights to hold, feed and cuddle her – or even to give her a bit of kangaroo care – if she is medically stable. There is no reason why the 24-hour light treatment cannot be interrupted for 30–60 minutes at a time, at least once a day, for this. You can also talk to or stroke your baby while she is under the lights (but perhaps not both, as this can be too much for premature babies). Let her know you are still there for her.

Usually babies undergoing phototherapy can carry on feeding as before. Although breast-milk can sometimes make the jaundice last longer, possibly because of the hormones it contains, you shouldn't be discouraged from feeding her your breast-milk if you've been able to make and/or express some – it's still the best food she could possibly have.

Outlook

Unless the jaundice has been very severe, it will clear up quickly with no harmful effects.

ANAEMIA

If your baby has anaemia it means that her blood does not have enough red blood cells. Red blood cells carry vital oxygen around the body; if there aren't enough of them, your baby's heart will have to pump harder to make the most of what oxygen is available. This makes her tired, and she may also have to breathe faster to get more oxygen. All babies, whether they are full term or premature, become slightly anaemic after they are born. In healthy term babies, this sorts itself out naturally within their first three or four months. Premature babies are more likely to need treatment, for two reasons.

First, a premature baby has missed the last weeks in the womb. Babies get most of the iron they need from their mothers in the last 12 weeks of pregnancy. Iron is essential

The smallest premature babies may only have 40ml (1½fl oz) of blood, compared with around 5 litres (8 pints) for the average adult woman. Because of the regular tests they need, a premature baby can lose the equivalent of what to you would be half a litre (a pint) of blood every week.

for making healthy red blood cells, and important for preventing anaemia. If your baby was born early she would have missed out on some, or perhaps all, of this.

The problem is compounded by the fact that they have so many blood tests. These are mostly routine ones, taken day after day: tests for blood gasses, blood glucose, haemoglobin count, electrolytes . . . The nurses take as little as possible each time, and hospital labs try to devise tests that only need tiny amounts of blood, but it still adds up. The amount of blood taken for each test varies from as much as 5ml when they are first admitted to the SCBU – this can be an eighth of a premature baby's entire supply – to as little as 0.2ml for a regular blood-gasses check. Most tests need nearer 1ml each, and they may in some cases have to be carried out two or three times every day.

There are some other possible causes too, but these are much less common than the two above. They include a mother and her baby having incompatible blood types or the mother bleeding before her baby was born, perhaps because her placenta was positioned over the exit from the womb (placenta praevia). There are also some infections that can trigger red blood cell breakdown.

If the anaemia comes on suddenly, your baby will be very obviously ill. She will look pale, have clammy skin and a fast pulse, and she will need extra oxygen. Tests can show that she has a low level of red blood cells and haemoglobin (the substance that does the actual oxygen-carrying, and makes blood red-coloured). If the anaemia comes on slowly you may notice that she gradually becomes less active (how easy it is to spot this depends on how active she was before) and that she looks pale and floppy. If she is feeding from a bottle or your breast she will seem to find this harder and more tiring. She may gain weight only slowly, or not at all, and she may also need extra oxygen.

Anaemia is not that much of a problem for a premature baby if it's mild and is effectively monitored and treated. However, if it is not spotted and becomes severe, it can cause serious breathing and heart problems.

Why can't I be my baby's blood donor?

Some parents, especially mothers, are very keen to give blood for any transfusions their baby may need. After all if you have grown your baby inside your own body, and may even now be feeding her on your breast-milk too, what could be more natural when she needs a life-saving blood donation, for you, or alternatively her father, to be the one who gives it, rather than some stranger? And in many countries using blood donated by parents is routine.

However, this is not possible in the UK at the moment, though some SCBUs are currently in negotiation with the National Blood Transfusion Service (NBTS). Doctors worry that you may have a low-level infection that you do not know about or that your blood groups may not be compatible, although technically either of these can be sorted out with a blood test.

The real difficulty is that there is a system at the NBTS that all donors' blood goes through, anonymously, for preparation and careful health/safety checks. And the service is just not – at the moment – geared up to handle a single blood donation from a specific person (you) and then ensure that it gets to a specific patient (your baby).

What staff may do to help

Your baby's doctors will do a blood test to check if her haemoglobin or red blood cell counts are low. Sometimes they don't need to do anything further except keep a sharp eye on the condition, so long as it is not making the baby unwell, because anaemia often rights itself in time.

If your baby's anaemia needs further investigation, they may do some more tests to check the size and shape of her red blood cells, look for any signs that the cells are being destroyed and check for any risk of bleeding in the baby herself. SCBU staff may well give your baby extra iron and folic acid too, but she will only need the folic acid until she reaches the day she should have been born; the

A nurse administering medication through an IV line.

iron can be stopped as soon as she is growing well and eating some solid food. (Iron may give your baby diarrhoea or constipation – and because it tastes unpleasant it needs to be disguised in her food or milk.)

For a time, your baby might also be given a weekly injection of a substance called erythropoietin, a chemical that the kidneys usually produce naturally. Premature babies' kidneys make this too, but not enough of it. Erythropoietin stimulates the bone marrow to make more red blood cells. If your baby is very unwell with anaemia, or if she is not yet too ill but her anaemia is gradually getting worse, she will be given a blood transfusion.

What parents can do

If you spend time just sitting beside and watching your baby, you will get to know what is normal behaviour for her and what is not, so you will notice any signs of anaemia or, if it has already been spotted, whether it is getting worse or better. Tell the nurses what you notice.

Outlook

Unless the anaemia was the result of some kind of a massive, uncontrolled blood loss, your baby will make a complete recovery, with no lasting ill effects.

INFECTIONS

Premature babies are especially vulnerable to infections. A premature baby's immune system has not yet had time to develop fully and grow strong, and because she was born early she has missed out on some of the infection-fighting antibodies she would usually have got from her mother, in the last three months of pregnancy. In addition, the necessary and life-saving treatments premature babies need to grow and survive often invade the baby's small body by breaking the skin barrier. Injections, heel prick tests, an IV line into her arm or leg or sometimes her scalp, vital equipment such as catheters or breathing or feeding tubes placed partially inside her body – all of these offer a possible way in for germs. Your baby may need several of these treatments and procedures at once, for days or even weeks. And each one carries a risk of infection with it.

Sepsis
Sepsis is the medical term for an infection – of any sort.

The commonest infection is probably septicaemia (a general infection of the blood, see over) followed by pneumonia, gut infections, skin infections around the umbilical cord area, urinary tract infections and meningitis.

There is information about some of these more severe infections on pages 57–81.

How can my baby get infected in hospital?

Your baby might have caught the infection before she was born. If you had the infection while you were pregnant, the infectious agent (bacteria, a virus or a fungus) might have crossed the placenta and entered your baby's body.

Some infections can be passed to a baby as she is being born, while she is travelling down the birth canal. And, if the waters break 24–48 hours before labour proper begins, because the barrier of the amniotic sac is torn, an infection can find a way through the tear in the membrane to reach the unborn baby.

However, your baby may well have caught the infection in hospital, from staff, visitors, equipment or other babies on the unit. Despite everyone's best efforts, even SCBUs can never be completely sterile places.

How infections arise

An infection develops when a germ (bacteria, a fungus or a virus) gate-crashes its way into a part of the body which can't fight it off, and multiplies there, causing pain or making you unwell. For instance, if you cut your finger and bacteria get in through the break in the skin, they will breed there, causing the area to swell, redden and hurt. But your body's immune system can usually contain the germs. This means the infection usually stays in your finger and doesn't spread to the rest of your body. An infection for a premature baby however usually entails more than a sore finger, because premature babies immune systems are not yet strong enough keep the germs trapped in the area where they first came in. So often the infection spreads, causing a general infection in the blood. This is a condition called septicaemia, which means 'infection of the blood'; it is sometimes called blood poisoning. If septicaemia is not spotted early enough and treated, it can make a premature baby very ill.

How to tell if your baby has an infection

It is sometimes hard to tell whether a premature baby has an infection. The signs may only be small and gradual, or they can be dramatic and show themselves fast. It depends on how severe the infection is, and what the cause is.

You might think that one of the most obvious signs would be a high temperature, as it is for a term baby, a child or an adult. It isn't. If anything a premature baby is more likely to be slightly chilly – hence some of the signs you see might be those of central cyanosis (see page 37) such as a bluish tinge to your baby's skin if she is Caucasian, or to the mucous membranes in her mouth if she is darker-skinned; or she may just have pale or mottled skin and chilly hands and feet.

She may have trouble with her breathing, perhaps breathing very fast (this is known as tachypnea), or with her chest sinking right in when she breathes, or even with long pauses between breaths. You may have difficulty with her feeding and she may have diarrhoea or vomiting. She may have seizures (see page 77), or be irritable, jittery and jumpy, or perhaps be listless and just generally seem unwell. There may be noticeable signs such as jaundice or spots, a rash, even discharge (perhaps from her eyes, nose or other infected area).

However, *all* these signs may be symptoms of other things too, and your baby may not have an infection at all.

Tests

If medical staff suspect an infection, they will take samples of your baby's blood, urine and perhaps spinal fluid too. These are given to the hospital lab to see if they can grow (culture) any bacteria, viruses or fungi from the samples. They may also test samples of mucus from your baby's nose or chest, or take a swab from any wound site to check for infections there. They may take X-rays of her chest or abdomen or make an ultrasound scan of her abdomen.

When Ben had an infection he was moved to an isolation ward, but he was not separated from his sister – she went along too.

Cough and cold caution

If you are the mother of a premature baby and have a mild cold, it is very unlikely that you would need to stay away from your own child unless she is either very unwell or extremely fragile and the staff advise it for a day or so. The good that you can do just being there beside her far outweighs the risk of her catching your germs. Newborn babies seldom seem to catch infections from their mothers anyway. However, anyone else – including father, brothers and sisters – should stay away from the baby if they have even the mildest sniff of a cold or other infection.

Even when a baby is sick and in a closed incubator, a loving parent can get very close.

What staff may do to help

To prevent infections, staff will wash their hands thoroughly when they first come into the SCBU and then should always wash their hands again or use alcohol hand-wipes after dealing with one baby and before going on to touch another. They should also follow strict hygiene rules for all equipment, and always be on the look-out for any signs of infection.

If an infection has already started, or doctors strongly suspect one, they will give your baby antibiotics immediately, without waiting for any test results. Premature babies are not yet strong and can become very ill very quickly, so doctors will usually give your baby broad-spectrum antibiotics (catch-all medication which tackles most general infections) right away, as lab results may take several days to come through. When they do get the results of the tests, they may change your baby's medication to give her one that targets her particular infection more specifically or more effectively.

What parents can do

Like the staff, you will be following strict hygiene rules, such as washing your hands thoroughly with medicinal soap and hot water whenever you come on to the unit to see your baby. Ask all your baby's visitors to do the same.

If your baby is ill with an infection, stay by her as much as you can, as your presence and love will help her tremendously. There are also many specific practical ways you can comfort your baby even if she is very sick or fragile, some without even touching her at all. (Please see the next chapter, *What can we do?*)

When it comes to telling whether your baby has an infection, you have a special advantage because, as her mother or father, you will probably know more about her than any of the staff, and you may instinctively know when your child is not herself. Neonatologists say that often parents will notice that something is wrong a good 24 hours before doctors are convinced. Typically, they say, parents usually notice first, then the nurses, who know the babies better than the doctors do, and lastly the doctors,

Shock

Shock is the medical term for the collapse of the blood circulation system.

Its effects include inadequate blood flow, not enough oxygen reaching the tissues and waste products not being removed properly from the blood. Symptoms include cold, sweaty, pale skin; a fast, weak pulse; a dry mouth; irregular breathing; and dilated pupils.

Shock can occur when a premature baby develops sepsis, suddenly loses a great deal of blood or has heart problems or even a severe allergic reaction.

because they are able to spend least time with any individual baby and know them least well.

This is especially likely if you have been able to spend time sitting beside her and just watching her, because you will have had the chance to absorb a good deal about her own special signs and body language (see page 86). You will also probably have been getting an increasingly good idea about what is normal for your baby, and what isn't. If she just does not seem quite right to you but you cannot put your finger on precisely why this is, tell a nurse you like and trust.

Outlook

Antibiotics usually clear up most bacterial infections completely and anti-fungal medications can be effective. There are only a few anti-viral drugs, so for many viral infections SCBUs must rely on 'supportive care' to increase the baby's ability to fight off the infection – this means giving the baby as much extra help as she needs with breathing, keeping her warm and comfortable, giving extra fluids to avoid dehydration and so on (they will give this supportive care to any sick baby, but will redouble their efforts for a baby with a viral infection).

Mild to moderate infections tend to leave no trace. But if an infection is severe it may cause other problems. In the short term, some release toxins (poisonous waste matter) into the blood; in addition to making your baby feel unwell, this can stop the blood clotting properly and so cause bleeding problems. If the infection interferes with a baby's blood pressure or the way her heart works, she may also go into shock (see left). It may also have altered the balance of certain vital substances, such as sodium, potassium, calcium or glucose, in the baby's blood. This can have harmful effects: for example too little/too much potassium can affect the way the heart works.

There are plenty of treatments for these complications. These include administering clotting agents, helping the baby's blood pressure to stay stable with extra fluids and medications, keeping her warm and well fed, giving her extra oxygen, using a ventilator, giving mild sedation to slow down the amount of oxygen she is using up and reducing her fluid intake or adding certain chemicals and substances to it.

Some severe infections may cause longer-term damage which takes time to heal properly. These infections are discussed in the next section.

SERIOUS MEDICAL PROBLEMS

Your premature baby may only have a few fairly minor health problems, which are easily treated, and then graduate relatively smoothly and quickly from her stay in the SCBU to going home with you. But some babies can have serious difficulties, punctuated by repeated setbacks. This section takes a look at some more serious disorders and at the many things that can be done about them.

This section may at first look a bit alarming – pages and pages giving details of one problem after another. However, it is not really meant to be read all the way through. Instead, you might like to use it by just turning to the particular relevant section if you'd like to find out more about a specific condition that your baby has, or one which she looks as if she may develop.

What you will find here is a basic factual account of each problem, its treatment and likely outcome, which you can use as a secure base for building up your own special knowledge about your baby's particular needs, using both the information from the neonatal staff about your baby's health and progress, and your own powerful instincts as her parents. This may make it is easier to ask the doctors and nurses the specific, informed questions that will give you the true picture of how your baby is doing.

WHAT PARENTS CAN DO

As the parents of a sick or very fragile premature baby you can be desperately anxious and may feel fearful and helpless. Many mothers and fathers whose premature babies have been ill say, however, that it helped them greatly to find out all they could about their baby's condition and treatment. It may help to write down all the

'There is no such thing as a bad question, or a question asked too often.'

Debbie Askin, Neonatal Nurse Practitioner, St Boniface General Hospital, Winnipeg questions you would like to ask on a small notepad you can carry with you easily – and their answers too. Ask a lot of questions, and ask them as many times as you need to. Experienced medical staff will expect this and understand.

Protecting and supporting your baby

There is a great deal that you as your baby's mother or father can do for your own child (even if you cannot physically pick her up and cuddle her), to comfort and protect her when she is very unwell, or to soothe her before and after an invasive investigation or operation. You also know or will come to know far more about your own baby than anyone else. If you would like some ideas or suggestions about supporting your baby, see the next chapter, *What can we do?*

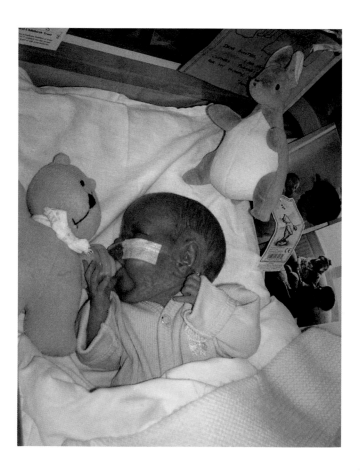

It can be disconcerting if your tiny baby begins to look fat and bloated. The most likely cause is a temporary build-up of fluid; the swelling will disappear when the fluid is drawn off.

RESPIRATORY DISTRESS SYNDROME (RDS)
Sometimes called HYALINE MEMBRANE DISEASE, or IDIOPATHIC RDS (IRDS)

Respiratory Distress Syndrome may develop if a baby's lungs are not mature enough or big enough to work properly, or if the baby is not making enough surfactant, the substance which usually coats the insides of the tiny air sacs in the lungs and stops them collapsing inwards. Without surfactant these air sacs (called alveoli), which make up the lungs, sag inwards between breaths. This makes it harder for the baby to take the next breath. A baby with RDS may have a real struggle to draw air down into her lungs. This can be exhausting, and it also means she is not getting enough oxygen. Fluid may then seep into the sacs, which makes it even more difficult for them to stay inflated with air.

The more prematurely a baby is born, the more likely she is to have this condition and the more severe it can be. About half of all the babies born at less than 30 weeks have RDS. In premature babies, making enough surfactant for their breathing to ease can be a slow process: the earlier a baby arrives, the slower the surfactant build-up, and the more help she will initially need with her breathing.

Symptoms

Neonatal staff can diagnose RDS by just looking at a baby, and seeing how she is breathing. Some babies show clear signs of RDS right from birth. The most obvious of these are the pulling in of the skin and muscles between or just below the ribs (retractions) as the baby tries to breathe, grunting, or panting as she breathes and the flaring of her nostrils as she tries harder to draw in air. She may also have bluish, dark red or mottled skin, or bluish membranes inside her mouth, showing that she's not getting enough oxygen, and apnoea spells.

Treatment

There is a very wide variation in how badly a premature baby may be affected by RDS. She may have it so mildly that the condition can safely be left to sort itself out without treatment. However, even if it is mild, the

Serious breathing problems

Of all the potentially serious problems a premature baby may have, breathing problems are the likeliest. Your baby's doctors will probably use respiratory distress syndrome as an umbrella term for breathing difficulties which have not been going on for long. If problems persist (become chronic) they tend to be referred to as chronic lung disease or broncho-pulmonary dysplasia (see page 60).

'Giving surfactant treatment automatically to all appropriate babies would save 1,400 premature babies' lives every year.'

Richard Cooke, Professor of Neonatal Medicine at Liverpool Women's Hospital

neonatal staff will still monitor her carefully to make sure all is well. If she has RDS more severely, a single dose of surfactant treatment (see below) is often enough to deal with it. But, sometimes, a baby's breathing difficulties are more acute and she will need breathing support (perhaps from CPAP or a mechanical ventilator; see page 30) and she may also need repeated surfactant treatments before she is better.

Surfactant treatment

Artificial surfactant fluid is given via a tube placed in the baby's windpipe. The thick liquid then drains gently down into her lungs. This is quite a specialized procedure and is most successful when it is carried out at a major SCBU where the staff are highly experienced in administering this particular treatment. As a back-up, a baby may also be given some extra air and oxygen using CPAP or a ventilator. According to Professor Halliday of Queen's University in Belfast, about 60 per cent of babies respond well to surfactant treatment, 30 per cent respond but slip back again and may need a second or even a third dose, and it does not really help the other 10 per cent.

The policy now in most major SCBUs is to give babies with RDS surfactant automatically, as if this is done the chances are they will not need any ventilation treatment at all. Babies can also be given surfactant at birth if they just look as if they might develop RDS, rather than waiting until they have already developed it.

Outlook

Mild cases often sort themselves out; less mild cases may only need a single dose of surfactant and be fine after that. Even severe cases have a good likely outcome, especially if surfactant treatment and additional breathing support are given promptly and correctly to the babies who need it.

However, if RDS becomes severe or is not treated properly, it can cause serious long-term breathing problems such as BPD, eye damage (retinopathy of prematurity), IVH, a heart problem called patent ductus arteriosus, or necrotizing enterocolitis (for these problems, see the entries that appear below).

BRONCHO-PULMONARY DYSPLASIA (BPD) CHRONIC LUNG DISEASE (CLD)

These are two different names for what is basically the same chronic (long-term) lung disorder. BPD/CLD is most often seen in premature babies who have had especial difficulty breathing and have therefore needed the help of artificial ventilator machines for several weeks to help them survive, although it also occurs in babies whose lungs have been damaged, for example by a pulmonary haemorrhage.

Your baby's being on a ventilator does not necessarily mean she will develop BPD. However, if these machines need to be used for long, they can damage premature babies' fragile lungs, causing BPD.

BPD can be very frustrating because it is something of a vicious circle. Very small or premature babies' lungs are often not mature enough or strong enough to cope with breathing air without some major help and they may need time on a ventilator. Yet the force at which ventilators push air into the windpipe can damage their fragile lungs, which will then find it even harder to work properly. This means a baby may possibly become dependent on the machine for her breathing – while her lungs continue to be damaged by the very device that is keeping her alive.

Symptoms

The damage to the lung itself involves scar tissue formation, which causes small areas of the lung to collapse altogether, while other areas trap air and balloon out. This is why, in X-rays, the lungs of a premature baby with BPD look bubbly.

BPD also affects the breathing tubes – the windpipe and tiny bronchioles in the lungs – causing them to produce too much mucus, which can clog them. It also causes twitchy, asthma-like spasms that interfere with breathing; in fact, if anyone in your family has asthma, this can also be a risk factor for a premature baby developing BPD.

Ventilators

Ventilators have made an enormous difference to the care of very sick premature babies since they were first used in the early 1970s, saving the lives of many thousands who would otherwise have died. Babies do not usually need a ventilator machine for long and most can be gradually weaned off it in less than a week.

Treatment

Chest X-rays will confirm whether or not your baby has BPD. She will need to be on a ventilator until she can breathe without it, but if possible staff will use an oscillatory or high-frequency ventilator (see page 33) as these are usually the gentlest on the lungs. Unfortunately not all hospitals have these, as they are very expensive. The SCBU will wean your baby off the ventilator very gradually. After this she will be supported with CPAP (see page 30) before finally graduating to breathing on her own.

Staff will also make sure your baby is getting extra calories, because she will be using a lot of energy, fighting to breathe if the machine allows her to take her own breaths in between ventilator 'breaths', and generally handling the stress of being constantly on a ventilator. She cannot breast- or bottle-feed, so she will have extra nourishment fed though a nasal tube or catheter. Staff may possibly give your baby some gentle chest physiotherapy, too. This can include delicately tapping her chest area with a finger or a tiny cup. However, this treatment is more usual in American hospitals than in British ones.

Medical staff may also, depending on your baby's needs, give her medicines. They could give her stimulants such as theophylline to stimulate her breathing, or sedatives and anti-anxiety drugs if she is becoming distressed by being on a ventilator. Diuretics may occasionally be used to help stop fluid collecting in her lungs. If she is in pain the staff may give her painkillers: either a short-acting drug such as fentanyl, or a longer-acting powerful one from the morphine family.

Coping with babies in distress

Babies can become distressed or agitated while they are on ventilators. It cannot be comfortable having a tube in your windpipe, often having no choice but to breathe with the rhythm of a machine rather than your own natural rhythm. They may also be in pain, or lying uncomfortably. Premature babies who have BPD can be especially sensitive to light, noise and being handled, and become exhausted very easily as the strain of being on a ventilator rapidly uses up all of the very little amounts of energy they have.

Ten weeks after his birth he is still scarcely bigger than his father's hand. He needs a nasal cannula to help him breathe and he is being fed through a naso-gastric tube. There is a long way to go. But he is out of the incubator and off the ventilator and father and son can find comfort in a cuddle.

Can my baby become addicted to painkillers?

Premature babies may well become temporarily physically dependent on drugs such as painkillers, sedatives or anti-anxiety medication if they have needed them for a while. Medical staff will therefore make very sure that any drugs like this will be tapered off slowly, never ever stopped suddenly.

If your baby has needed to have this type of medication for a couple of weeks or more, talk to her nurses about whether physical dependence might be a problem for her. If they feel this is possible, ask them how she is going to be weaned off her medication when the time is right.

According to Dr Kathleen VandenBerg, of the Children's Hospital in Oakland, California, they may also have the sense of fear that can come from being 'air hungry' or unsure about their breathing capacity.

One answer to this agitation and distress is sedatives. These will calm a baby down; but if she is in pain, these drugs may also give the baby's carers the impression that she is content, when she is not. In fact one study (see *References*) suggests that sedative drugs may actually make babies more sensitive to pain, not less. Anti-anxiety drugs, too, can make a baby more peaceful but may mask pain.

However, babies who have BPD are not easy to comfort. They can be hard to bond with or relate to as they are so often stressed, agitated and exhausted. This can be difficult for parents trying to get close and give love to their babies. Your baby may tend to squirm and arch herself away if you try to hold her, or simply turn away or shut her eyes because, in her distress, she cannot even cope with her parents' faces trying to make loving contact with her. This can be really disheartening, enough to make even the sanest and most competent, calm and loving mother or father feel helpless and inadequate.

If your baby has BPD and is behaving in this way, try to remember that it is not you she is rejecting. It's more likely that she is finding the situation she is in too much to cope with, and trying to handle it in the only way she can – perhaps by trying to shut everything out or pulling away from any other form of stimulation, like a cuddle, your voice or your face. But she does need you badly. She needs to feel your presence beside her and she needs your love, your help, your support and protection in ways that she can cope with. See the chapter *What can we do?* for some ideas that may help.

Outlook

A baby or child with BPD who has the right constant care will get better, even though she may be anything from three months to six years old before her breathing is totally problem-free. She will need to be weaned away from the ventilator, or from extra oxygen help, slowly and gradually; she may still need extra oxygen while feeding from your breast or a bottle for a while. A very few babies who are otherwise well will go home with oxygen equipment and continue their therapy at home to help their lungs carry on strengthening and healing. (See the section on caring for babies who need extra oxygen for a while at home in *Time to go home*, page 169.)

An IV line provides a vital channel for medication or fluids. Bound to the baby's arm, a splint helps to hold the line secure.

PATENT DUCTUS ARTERIOSUS (PDA)

When a baby is still developing in the womb, he or she has a short passageway or duct called the *ductus arteriosus* (DA) linking two of the big blood vessels leaving the heart. In an unborn baby, the DA links the main artery supplying the body, called the aorta, with another big artery, the pulmonary artery, which takes blood from the heart to the lungs. This passageway is meant to close up soon after she is born. But in some newborns, usually babies born

65

PDA is one of the most common heart problems for premature babies. Around one in five of premature babies who weigh less than 1,500g (3lb 5oz) when they are born has PDA.

prematurely, this small connecting passageway either stays open; or closes, then opens back up again. When this happens, it is called *patent* (open) *ductus arteriosus*.

While this duct stays open babies do get enough oxygen, but their lungs may get too much blood to cope with. This can cause some serious side-effects, especially if the baby is very premature, such as fluid gathering in her lungs or, if her lungs stop working properly, becoming (and then possibly remaining) dependent on an artificial ventilator. The good news is that PDA often sorts itself out with time, and it may be so mild that it causes your baby little or no problem at all.

However, if a baby is very unwell or fragile she will not be able to afford to wait for the condition to correct itself and she will need treatment for the PDA before it starts causing complications.

Symptoms

PDA is usually diagnosed from the sound of your baby's heart heard through an ordinary stethoscope; the doctor may be able to hear the 'continuous murmur' sound that it makes. Other signs include the baby's blood-pressure reading, any trouble she may be having with her breathing or if she has an unusually powerful pulse which may be seen or felt anywhere – in the groin, wrist or top of the foot, for example. PDA can be confirmed by an X-ray of the heart or a Doppler ultrasound scan (a type of scan that can show movement) to check how the blood flows throughout the heart.

Treatment

The treatment the doctors decide on will depend on how big the PDA opening is, and how much difficulty it is causing. If it is not too serious, they will try reducing the amount of fluids in your baby's body. Usually a diuretic medicine (one that will make her urinate out excess fluid) will be tried first and this is often successful.

However, if your baby also has another condition, such as jaundice, which may be made worse by this type of medication, or if the PDA is more serious, they may decide to do an operation to repair it: with the baby under a general anaesthetic, a surgeon will close the PDA with a clip or a surgical stitch. This takes about an hour and babies usually do well afterwards. Following her operation your baby will probably have a small tube draining any air away from her chest for a couple of days until the area begins to heal.

Outlook

Babies usually do well after their PDA closes or has been closed. However this heart condition can sometimes be a risk factor for long-term breathing problems.

NECROTIZING ENTEROCOLITIS (NEC)

A potentially serious condition which affects the bowels of some newborn babies, necrotizing enterocolitis can occur when something is interfering with the blood flow to the

Born at 24 weeks, in his first week of life John survived a pulmonary haemorrhage and a cardiac arrest, and then developed necrotizing enterocolitis. He is now a healthy three-year-old (see the photograph on pages 174-5).

Breast-milk helps to protect babies against developing NEC.

baby's bowel, causing the area to die and then become infected.

NEC can be so mild that it can be cured simply by stopping feeds by mouth for your baby for a week or so and using IV feeding instead, to give the bowel a rest. However, at the other end of the scale, NEC can become severe enough to rupture the bowel wall and cause a serious infection called peritonitis in the abdominal cavity.

Premature babies are particularly vulnerable to NEC because they have immature digestive systems and a tendency to developing problems which stop their blood taking oxygen round their body efficiently. There is no single cause of NEC, but anything which affects the smooth flowing of your baby's blood can lead to asphyxia (too little oxygen getting to her tissues) and therefore to NEC. Risk factors include sepsis, repeated apnoea spells, not having grown very well in the womb, the bowel not forming normally, low blood pressure, cold, stress, patent ductus arteriosis or moderate to severe bradycardia.

Symptoms

Babies with NEC can have a wide variety of symptoms, some of which can be quite subtle. This is why parents, who know their own baby better than anyone, may notice there is something not quite right even before the neonatal staff do. Important obvious signs are a bloated tummy and small amounts of blood in your baby's bowel movements. She may be vomiting, her feed may stay in her stomach for longer than usual, or she might just be generally off-colour, not wanting to feed and seeming tired and listless; and her temperature may be (even) less steady than usual. If your baby has severe NEC she will be very ill or listless, with a taut tummy and show signs of being in pain. Sometimes babies' limbs will also be swollen.

Since it can be difficult to tell for sure whether a baby has NEC, the doctors will probably order X-rays to check for any swellings in your baby's bowel or for the tell-tale gas bubbles. They would probably also check how much milk is getting left behind in your baby's stomach after feeds and test her bowel movements for traces of blood.

Treatment

The medical staff will stop your baby having any feeds by mouth. Instead, they will feed her either intravenously, or by using a tube that passes straight into her gut below the site of the NEC, for up to a week or sometimes even longer. This will give the affected part of her bowel a rest from food and time to heal. They may also give antibiotics in case an infection has started and may put in a drain to take away any mucus that may have formed.

When feeds are introduced again, your baby should have breast-milk, if possible, instead of formula milk. Breast-milk is much easier to digest, and contains enzymes and other special substances which can have a healing effect on the gut lining itself. If giving breast-milk is not possible, there is a special low-allergy milk formula which may be used instead.

Because a baby with NEC can become very ill quite rapidly she needs a close eye kept on her. This means she may have frequent X-rays, sometimes twice a day, to check that the bowel wall has not ruptured. She might also need some extra oxygen or ventilation in case of apnoea or shock, and perhaps some extra fluids and medication to keep her blood pressure steady.

Surgery and its consequences

A baby with mild NEC will usually start to improve after a few days of antibiotics and IV feeding. However, if she does not start getting better pretty promptly or if there are signs that there is a bowel problem that might need to be repaired with surgery, her specialist may do an operation to look inside her gut to see what is happening.

Even if a baby has responded to treatment and recovered, she may still need surgery. Sometimes a baby's bowel can narrow around the NEC site as the area heals and produces scar tissue. Gut inflammation can also cause internal scarring. Either may create a blockage or narrowing in a baby's gut, though this can be put right quite easily with an operation.

Most seriously, if your baby's bowel has ruptured she will need emergency surgery to try to correct the problem

Milk banks

If you cannot give your own breast-milk, it may be possible to get some from a breast-milk bank. At the time of writing, there are 14 of these special hospital milk banks in the UK, and they will also give milk to other hospitals' SCBUs when they can.

Short gut syndrome

Occasionally, so much of the bowel is affected by NEC and has to be removed that there is not enough left to absorb food, and it may be some time before the baby can take all her feeds by mouth once again. Until she can, she will be fed via an IV line (see page 26).

by removing the damaged or scarred section of the bowel. Your baby may come back from theatre with an ostomy – a narrow, open passageway from the bowel which ends in a small opening on the abdomen's surface called a stoma. The stoma has a small collection bag fitted carefully over it which collects the baby's stools (faeces). If the opening has been made into the large intestine it is called a **colostomy**; if it leads out from the small intestine, it is called an **ileostomy**. Both of these rest the lower part of the gut from its usual job of processing food and waste matter, and allow it more time to heal and grow.

Your baby's surgeon will carry out a second operation later on to join the ends of the now-healed-up bowel back together, and close up the stoma again.

Outlook

Good. Around three-quarters of babies with NEC get better just by being treated with antibiotics and having no feeds by mouth for a week. The problem sometimes recurs and the treatment has to be repeated. If a baby has surgery, this is usually successful. However, severe NEC is a very serious illness, and can sometimes be fatal.

If, after an operation to remove the damaged section, your baby's gut is now too short to be able to absorb enough nutrition from her food, she may need extra IV feeding, special milk formula and supplements for some months to make sure she is getting enough nutrients to grow healthy and strong. The gut will usually re-grow sufficiently to function properly but very occasionally an ostomy needs to be permanent.

INTRA-VENTRICULAR HAEMORRHAGE (IVH)

Babies are usually only at risk of IVH in their first 2–3 days of life. However, an existing IVH 'bruise' can get bigger for a few days after it forms. If a baby is three days old (or more) and has not had an IVH yet, he or she is very unlikely to have one.

Any bleeding into the natural spaces in the brain, the ventricles, is called an intra-ventricular haemorrhage. Though this sounds worrying, it is very common in preterm babies, and it is usually so slight that, were it not for the routine brain scans carried out on very premature newborn babies, no one would ever know it had happened. The baby's system will tend to reabsorb any IVH blood naturally over the first few weeks, just as the blood from a bruise is absorbed back into your body.

IVH tends to happen because premature babies have a very rich blood supply to their brains, but this blood mostly flows through quite fragile capillaries. When the baby is being born, the strength of the blood flow and amount of oxygen reaching her brain changes many times, and may cause some of the weaker capillaries to break open and leak blood. Other possible causes can include anything which produces a major change in the brain's blood flow, such as severe BPD (see page 60).

Although IVH is generally harmless, occasionally it can be serious. Sometimes the bleeding may make the brain ventricles expand. Though that, too, often clears up leaving no trace that it has ever happened, it can have some longer-term side-effects. For instance, there may be

A naso-gastric tube carries his food through his nose, down his throat to his stomach.

Hydrocephalus

Hydrocephalus is a condition in which the normal flow of cerebro-spinal fluid around the brain is blocked (an IVH can cause such a blockage). The fluid builds up in the ventricles of the brain, which makes them swell.

Hydrocephalus is sometimes referred to as water on the brain.

Lumbar puncture

A procedure for removing some of the cerebro-spinal fluid – the fluid that circulates around the spine and brain. This is kept inside a membrane which covers both brain and spinal column. A needle is passed gently into the lumbar region – the area at the base of the spine – piercing the membrane and drawing off some of the fluid.

some bleeding within the tissue of the brain itself (this is called *haemorrhagic parenchymal infarction*). Again, a baby may show no sign of this at the time, but the brain cells die in the area where the haemorrhage occurred, leaving an empty space or cyst. Another possibility is that fluid may build up in the ventricles and cause them to swell.

Luckily, a cyst caused by IVH usually clears up of its own accord and any swelling dies away again. If so, the baby may well be none the worse for her IVH. However, in some cases premature babies may develop more serious difficulties such as cerebral palsy (see page 78), problems with their hearing or their sight, or learning difficulties. Severe IVH can be fatal.

Symptoms

If a baby does have more serious IVH, it can cause symptoms that may include apnoea, bradycardia, anaemia, seizures, floppiness and lethargy. The soft spot (called the fontanelle) on the top of her head may also bulge.

A diagnosis of IVH will be confirmed by an ultrasound scan of the baby's head. This procedure can be done at her bedside if need be.

Treatment

Usually no treatment is needed for IVH. However, if fluid is building up in the ventricles, some of the extra fluid can be removed using a lumbar puncture, so reducing the swelling. Alternatively, staff may give your baby medication which slows down the amount of fluid being made, again reducing the swelling.

Occasionally an IVH can cause build-up of fluid in the brain (hydrocephalus, see above) that does not clear either on its own or with medication. In these cases, the baby will have an operation to insert a small tube called a shunt, which removes the fluid as it is being made. This slim tube runs from the brain – going in just behind the ear – down under her skin to her abdomen, where the fluid is reabsorbed again.

A shunt is not nearly as cumbersome or noticeable as it sounds. When the baby develops more fat under her skin and grows more hair you cannot even see the tube.

Sometimes the shunt may be temporary, but usually it will need to be permanent.

If the haemorrhage caused a good deal of blood to be diverted from her body's usual supply, your baby may be given a blood transfusion. If the IVH was a major one, the baby will probably have special physiotherapy and support to reduce its effects. Babies who have had anything other than a very mild IVH need to have a special hearing test while they are still on the SCBU.

9 out of 10 IVHs sort themselves out with few – or no – long-term problems at all.

Outlook

If your baby has had an IVH which was marked enough to be noticed by her doctors, she will be followed up as an out-patient of the hospital with regular check-ups, so that any long-term problems which might possibly be developing can be spotted early, and the treatments which would be the most helpful begun as soon as possible.

Developmental milestones Parents and doctors assess how a baby's development is coming along by seeing when the baby reaches specific developmental milestones such as smiling, sitting without help, crawling, walking, saying her first words. If it does turn out that there is a problem, it may respond well to physiotherapy, speech therapy or special learning schemes.

Movement and muscle tone problems After an IVH a baby's movements can be jerkier and less well co-ordinated and her muscle tone can be too tense or too floppy. Movement or posture problems like this are often labelled as cerebral palsy (CP, see page 78) but they usually improve so much that they disappear on their own as the baby gets older. This is why a diagnosis of CP is tricky and cannot safely be made until a child is 12–18 months old, unless the CP is very severe. If muscle tone and control problems do not sort themselves out, they can usually be helped by physiotherapy.

Sight and hearing Some babies may develop sight or hearing problems (though most premature babies' hearing difficulties are not anything to do with IVH). If your baby has had an IVH she should have her hearing checked around the time she goes home. It is also possible that her vision may be slightly affected. The most common result is some form of squint, which can usually be put right by the hospital's eye specialists.

Seizures After a major IVH, a baby may occasionally have seizures – also commonly called fits or convulsions (see page 77) – for several months, even after she is well enough to go home. These can be treated successfully with drug therapy.

Hydrocephalus If your baby has a shunt to treat her hydrocephalus, this may sometimes become blocked, disconnected or cause an infection. Parents get to know the problem signs very quickly. An infection causes a temperature or reddening skin over the area where the shunt is, and if the tube is blocked or has disconnected, a baby may be abnormally sleepy, have jerkier movements, be especially irritable or have fits. If you are at all concerned, take your child to hospital for a check-up; most potential problems can be stopped in their tracks by swift treatment. (Please see *Helplines*, page 203, for details of the Hydrocephalus Association if you would like to find out any more specific details about this.)

The retina

The retina is a delicate ten-layer covering of special light-sensitive nerve cells coating the back of the eye. It registers the images that your eyes see and sends them flashing down the optic nerve, which runs from the retina to the brain, where they are 'officially' recognized.

RETINOPATHY OF PREMATURITY (ROP)

ROP is a disorder of the retina of the eye which usually only affects babies who are born at less than 32 weeks. Up to 30 per cent of extremely premature babies (less than 28 weeks gestational age) will develop it to some degree. This is because though babies' eyes begin to form after only four weeks inside the womb, their retinas do not start developing until 28 weeks or so. Because eyes are the last sense organs to become complete, they are especially vulnerable to damage in babies who are born early.

How does ROP happen?

When the retina develops normally, it begins to grow a delicate, spiders'-web network of tiny blood vessels, which starts at the centre of the retina and spreads slowly outwards. This process is finished a week or so after a baby is born, if she has gone to term. However, when a baby arrives prematurely, the retina's blood vessels do not have the chance to finish developing in the peace and dim light of the womb, and have to do so in a harsher, usually brightly lit, environment instead.

If a baby develops ROP, this steady, symmetrical growth pattern – which looks like the fine, filigree roots of a new plant – is disrupted. The blood capillaries begin to grow too fast, and untidily. This can cause bleeding inside the eye and the formation of scar tissue, which pulls at the delicate retina. In severe cases, the retina comes away from the back of the eye altogether. This is rare, but it does sometimes happen; the condition is known as retinal detachment and means the baby will be partially blind.

There is no simple explanation for why these blood vessels develop oddly, but one of the main reasons seems to be too-high levels of oxygen in the baby's bloodstream. Premature babies' systems are geared towards having exactly the right amount of oxygen to suit them at every stage of their development. In the womb, this perfect amount is delivered directly into a baby's bloodstream via the placenta and her own umbilical cord. However, if a baby is born early, both her breathing and her regulatory systems may be too immature to make sure she absorbs the right amount of oxygen from whatever breathing method she is suddenly having to use – whether she is breathing in oxygen from the surrounding air naturally or having artificial help.

This may mean either that the baby can take in too much oxygen, or that she has trouble regulating the levels of it in her bloodstream. If she is getting too much oxygen, this may encourage the vulnerable newly forming blood vessels in the retina to grow in a disorganized way. There are several risk factors for ROP which make sense if the too-much or fluctuating oxygen theory is true, including apnoea, repeated blood transfusions, unstable blood pressure, IVH, patent ductus arteriosus, infections and multiple pregnancy (being one of twins, triplets or more).

Checking your baby's eyes

If your baby was born before she had spent 32 weeks in the womb, she should have her eyes checked routinely by an

Some research suggests that bright light might cause eye damage in premature babies. SCBUs are usually brightly lit by fluorescent tubing; in fact, in most SCBUs the lighting has actually become five to ten times brighter over the past 20 years. Yet in the womb, babies are in protective semi-darkness.

In the US, hospitals now tend to shade premature babies' eyes from glare, although in the UK only a few units do this at the moment.

eye specialist (ophthalmologist) every month or so to make sure the blood vessels in her retinas are developing normally. If there are any signs of ROP, the specialist will assess how mild or serious it is and how it is progressing, and will give whichever treatment is needed.

The eye examination is not thought to hurt, but it looks pretty uncomfortable. Some parents prefer to stay and soothe their baby while it is being carried out. Others feel they would rather not watch but make sure they are there immediately afterwards to help settle their baby once again. The ophthalmologist uses eye drops to enlarge the baby's pupils so he can shine a light throughout them to see the retina behind. He also uses an instrument called a lid retractor to hold the eye open, plus another to push down gently on the white of the eye.

Treatment

Because ROP usually gets better of its own accord, your baby may not need any treatment, although doctors will keep a regular check on how her eyes are developing. If the ROP has progressed, it may need some minor surgery.

This may involve **cryotherapy**, which freezes the abnormal blood vessels to stop them growing. Cryotherapy is done with a tiny probe and liquid nitrogen as the freezing agent, under either a local or a general anaesthetic. Your baby's eyes will be swollen for a few days afterwards, but soothing ointments, eyedrops and cold compresses can all help. So might homeopathic arnica – but check with your baby's doctors and a medically qualified homeopath (see *Helplines*, page 203).

The other method is **laser treatment**, which uses a tiny, powerful light beam to destroy the abnormal blood vessels. This treatment can be done under a light anaesthetic, so there will be less of an anaesthesia 'hangover' afterwards, and it also causes less discomfort and swelling. Lasers for ROP are still being tested out in several different hospitals world-wide.

Outlook

For around three-quarters of babies with mild ROP, there is no scarring or damage to the eyes. Some mild cases, however, do result in minor vision problems: these may mean that the child will need glasses – for short-sightedness, for example – or treatment with minor surgery and an eye-patch for crossed eyes (strabismus) or 'lazy eye' (amblyopia).

Normal jittery movements tend to stop if you place your hand gently on the baby's back, or cup her head and feet lightly; seizures don't.

SEIZURES

Also known as fits or convulsions, seizures happen when the brain's electrical systems short-circuit. A seizure is usually a sign that something is either irritating, or has damaged, the brain. Many babies who have seizures will only experience them mildly and briefly, but some have severe attacks again and again.

A seizure may happen because of an infection; because of imbalances in the usual substances found in the blood (for example low blood sugar or low calcium levels); after a major IVH or swelling of the brain (see hydrocephalus, page 72 and IVH, page 70), or as a consequence of shortage of oxygen or brain malformation. When no one can find out what is causing them, they are called idiopathic seizures.

Symptoms

The most obvious signs of a seizure are jerking movements of the body, stiffening of the arms, arching the back and flickering movements in the eyes, eyelids, mouth or tongue. There may be episodes of frantic sucking or apnoea and/or bradycardia. Afterwards the baby may be especially tired or sleepy for anything from a few minutes to a few hours.

However, diagnosing a seizure can be tricky, because premature babies' movements are usually jerky until their nervous systems have matured. To check for seizures the doctors may have to carry out various tests. An electro-encephalogram (EEG) will check out the electrical activity in your baby's brain. An ultrasound scan of the brain will show if there is any IVH swelling, or perhaps a malformation which could have caused the problems.

For a more accurate picture, a CT (computerized tomography) scan or an MRI (magnetic resonance imaging) scan may be carried out instead. Staff may also test your baby's blood or spinal fluid to see if there is an infection.

Treatment

If your baby is having seizures, she will be given anticonvulsant medicine, such as phenobarbitone, which also acts as a calming sedative. However, this can cause lowered blood pressure and less easy breathing so staff should keep a careful watch on both.

Outlook

It is important to stress that most babies do recover completely from seizures and have no long-term ill effects. However, if the seizures happened because of severe oxygen shortage or a disease of the brain itself, they can continue to occur over a long period of time, and may be associated with a degree of brain damage. But whether this damage is caused by the oxygen shortage or brain disease or by the convulsions, no one is quite sure.

If your baby has had repeated moderate-to-severe seizures, she will need regular follow-up visits to a neurologist or neonatologist to check her progress.

CEREBRAL PALSY (CP)

Cerebral palsy jumbles the messages that flash between the brain and muscles. If a child has CP, her brain is not controlling the muscles in the normal way. This may be because part of the brain is not working in the right way, perhaps because it has been destroyed or has not developed properly.

Although in many cases there is no obvious reason for cerebral palsy, there are various possible causes. These include severe shortage of oxygen, perhaps as a result of a difficult or premature birth, IVH, or an infection during the first few weeks when the baby was developing inside the mother (such as German measles). Very occasionally, CP may be caused by a rare genetic disorder. This can be inherited, even if neither parent has CP.

Symptoms

Initially, it is very hard to tell whether a premature baby has cerebral palsy, since between 40 and 80 per cent of

There are three main types of cerebral palsy (CP):

1 **Spastic CP**, in which the child's muscles are stiff and it is harder for her to move her joints

2 **Athetoid CP**, in which the muscles change from being floppy to being tense in a way the child cannot control,; she may also have speech and hearing problems

3 **Ataxic CP**, in which lack of control makes it difficult for the child to balance, and often causes jerky movement and speech

babies born early and weighing less than 1,600g (3½lb) do not have ordinary muscle tone or reflexes anyway at first. Jerky movements and poor muscle tone and posture are common in premature babies, but these problems have usually sorted themselves out by the time the child is 12 to 18 months old.

True CP only affects 3–6 per cent of premature babies. Any problems a baby may have with movement or muscle control that look as if they might possibly be CP will need to be closely monitored for between 6 and 18 months before a paediatrician can be certain either way. The less severe the cerebral palsy is, the longer it takes to diagnose.

Usually it is the lower part of the baby's body that is affected. This can cause difficulties with balancing, sitting, walking and crawling, and also sometimes stiffness and muscle tightness in the legs. The intelligence of a baby

A sensor pad on the baby's foot monitors the level of oxygen in his blood.

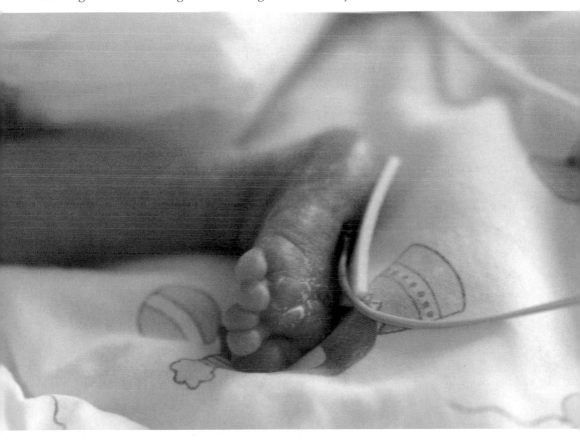

with CP may be completely normal (and sometimes well above average) but, as they grow older, some may have learning difficulties.

Treatment

Treatment includes physiotherapy to help your baby's muscle development and posture. If babies' muscles are too stiff to work with, doctors may prescribe a drug called baclofen to relax the muscles. In some cases a baby with CP may also have an operation to correct any muscle tightness or contraction or any shortening of the muscles and ligaments that has developed, if these cannot be improved by exercise alone. For children who develop learning difficulties, there is a range of teaching methods which can be enormously helpful (see *Helplines,* page 203).

Outlook

The effects of CP can vary very widely, from the barely noticeable to the severely debilitating. If you want to know more about the likely effects as your baby grows, see pages 186–8. If you would like further specific information about CP, or just a listening ear, talk to your baby's nurse, paediatrician or neonatologist or to SCOPE's helpline (see page 203).

SERIOUS INFECTIONS

Some infections can arise as complications of a premature baby's illnesses or health problems. Two of the most serious are pneumonia and meningitis.

Pneumonia

Pneumonia is an acute infection of the lungs.

Symptoms Signs that your baby has a serious lung infection include difficulty in breathing or a change in the way she usually breathes, fluid in her lungs and an increasing number of apnoea spells. To confirm pneumonia, the doctor will use a stethoscope to listen for the sound of fluid in your baby's lungs, and take an X-ray or perhaps extract a small sample of lung fluid via a tube so that the hospital lab can check for infection.

Treatment Your baby will be given a course of antibiotics (about five days long on average) either by IV or by injection. She may also have some extra oxygen, special nutrition and temperature control, and she might need support from a ventilator.

Outlook If pneumonia is spotted early and treated promptly, premature babies have an excellent chance of recovering completely. If not, it may lead to permanent lung damage or other serious infections such as meningitis.

Meningitis

This is an infection or inflammation of the membranes covering the spinal cord or brain (the meninges). The infection may be viral or bacterial in origin.

Symptoms These can include many that are not unique to this illness, such as a baby having an increased number of apnoea spells, a fluctuating heart and/or breathing rate, going off her feeds, arching her back and a tense fontanelle area. Doctors will confirm a diagnosis of meningitis by taking a small sample of her spinal fluid via a lumbar puncture (see page 72) for examination in the hospital lab.

Treatment Staff will give her antibiotics if the infection is bacterial and she may need extra intensive care, including ventilator support and extra oxygen, intubated nutrition and extra fluids and, if possible, round-the-clock, one-to-one nurse observation.

Outlook Usually the infection is spotted early and treated promptly, and babies make a good recovery. But if the treatment is not very successful meningitis can result in brain and nervous system complications. It also depends what type of meningitis it is as to how useful antibiotics are.

If a baby has had severe seizures or been in a coma, there is a possibility of brain damage or even death.

What can
we do?

'I watched them for a while. They all looked like they knew just what they were doing. I felt so shaky and upset that I couldn't see what there might be for me to do too. So I just sat by Sacha.'

Julie, mother of Sacha, born at 33 weeks

Many parents say that when they first came into the high-tech SCBU and saw their babies surrounded by machinery and being cared for by busy, efficient neonatal nurses they felt intimidated, and almost as if they had been left out.

It may sometimes feel as though, because the nurses and doctors have taken charge of caring for your baby and seem to be doing it all so well, there is little you can really do to help. This could not be further from the truth. Just how hands-on you can be depends on how well your baby is, but there is an enormous amount both mothers and fathers can do every day, even for the most fragile of premature babies, and even while they are still in hospital.

STAFF AND PARENTS TOGETHER

Neonatal staff and parents can make a great team. This is because you can do vital things for your baby that the nurses cannot, and the nurses and doctors can help your baby in ways that you cannot.

Your baby already knows you

Parents' natural confidence can be shaken to its foundations by the shock of a premature birth, and a baby who may be unwell, and need special care. Many cannot believe that they already have their own special connections with their small son or daughter. And the barriers of special care, such as closed incubators, monitor leads and machinery, can make even the most confident mother or father feel cut off from their child. But if you are his mother, your baby has until very recently been physically sharing your body. Research shows that while babies are in their mothers' wombs, mother and baby are so closely connected that the baby can even be aware of his mother's moods.

Mothers are the people that new babies know best in the world. It may sound odd to say your baby already knows you, especially if at the moment he is very premature or unwell and it seems as if he is not responding much to anything, even when you sit beside him or talk to him. Yet your baby already knows *your* voice. He will have been born knowing it because he has spent many hours hearing you talk, laugh, sing and shout while you carried him inside your womb. The sound may have been muffled but it was yours and so it is your voice that has more power to comfort and reassure him than anyone else's.

Why your baby needs you

Mothers and fathers can give their baby their undivided attention, protection and care. You are the only people who are there entirely for your baby or babies: nurses' care has to be shared. You are the one constant factor in your baby's life.

And mothers can make breast-milk. This is so good for premature babies that it amounts to a valuable part of their medical treatment (see page 69).

Working together to support your baby

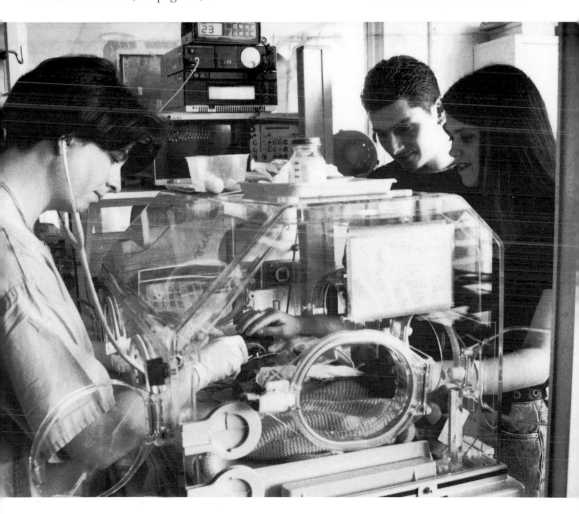

Nurses change at every shift: parents don't.

'Trust yourself. You know more than you think you do.'

Dr Benjamin Spock

When your baby

★ has a bright, shiny alert look in his eyes

★ is making 'ooh' shapes with his mouth

★ can pay attention – perhaps only for a few seconds – to something such as your face, a moving toy, your voice

★ is trying to lift his head or turn, as you hold him against your shoulder

he is happy and may be ready for some interaction with you

More importantly, you are the only people who can give your baby love: you can comfort and soothe him and give him your time. In fact parents are their baby's best comforters – just being there for him can have a positive effect on his health. Neonatal staff say that they have often seen the level of oxygen in premature babies' systems rise when their mothers or fathers came to sit beside them, even though the babies had not opened their eyes nor the parents said a word.

You are also the ones who know your baby best. It may not seem so at first, but when you have spent more time with your baby you will find that – despite all the medical expertise surrounding him – this is true. This is partly because you have the time to spend sitting by him and watching him day after day: nurses do not have the time to do this. Because of this, you are usually the first to know if your baby is unwell or if he is getting better, and whether he is comfortable, coping with what is happening to him or getting distressed. You are also your baby's best advocates and protectors. All this makes a great difference to how well he is cared for.

BABYWATCHING: UNDERSTANDING YOUR BABY'S SIGNALS

One of the most important – and most natural – things you can do is to understand your baby. Many parents say they feel helpless, especially if their baby is very unwell, and all they can do is just sit by his incubator, but this is the perfect place to be to get to know your baby – the better to understand his own personal signals and body language.

You may think that because your baby is not yet mature enough to cry or smile you will not be able to understand what he is feeling. Yet even though he has been born too early and his body is very small, he is sending you many different, definite messages. He can do this without crying, without words, sometimes without even moving.

All babies, including premature babies, use body language and facial expressions to tell you how they are or what they need. This is not an exact language, but it offers valuable clues to what your baby is feeling. And as almost any neonatal nurse will tell you, it's usually you – your baby's mother or father – who can read your own baby the best, partly because you are his parent, and partly because you spend far more time sitting beside him and watching over him than anyone else.

There is no such thing as a definitive guide to the way premature babies communicate. Each baby is a unique individual and the meaning of the signals your baby gives you depends a good deal on how many weeks he spent in the womb before he was born and how mature, and how well, he is at the moment. It can also depend on how he is being cared for, what medication he is having (some types can have a sedating effect) or whether he is on a ventilator.

Some signals can have different meanings at different times. As you watch them, try to think what – knowing, as only you do, your baby's particular and special

'You cannot say a newborn baby does not talk. It is we who do not listen.'

Frederick Leboyer, obstetrician and natural childbirth pioneer

When your baby brings his hand up to his face it is a good sign. He is able to comfort himself without waiting for you to do it for him.

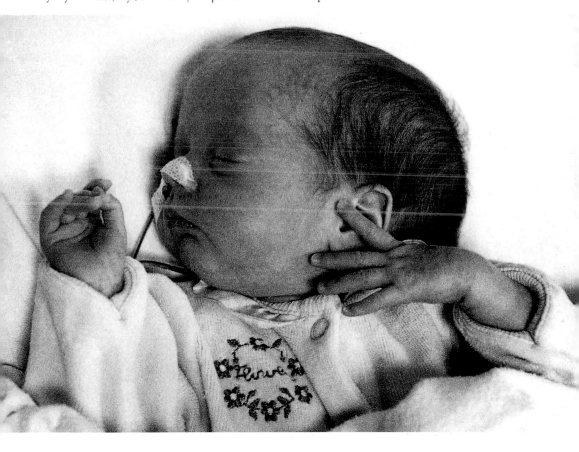

When your baby

★ is lying with his arms and legs relaxed

★ looks alert, his eyes open and shiny

★ has a smooth, relaxed face – not taut, no lines or furrows

★ has tried to curl himself over sideways

★ has pink, even skin colour

(And, in a more mature premature baby –)

★ is looking at you, or at something, with interest (rather than staring fixedly)

★ may be trying to smile

he's showing that he's feeling comfortable

When your baby tries or manages to

★ clasp his hands together

★ bring his hands up to or near his mouth or face

★ suck on his fingers or hands

★ hold on to the corner of his blanket

★ have his feet touching, one on top of the other

★ tuck himself into a cosy, curled-over position

★ turn his gaze or head away

he's showing he can comfort himself

circumstances – they might mean. If your baby yawns or hiccups, for instance, this may be a way of breaking away from something that is happening to him because he can no longer cope with it, or it may mean that he is becoming slightly short of oxygen. Or, of course, a yawn may simply mean that he is tired.

Interpreting the clues

All the signs need a bit of interpreting. It may take a parent or an expert neonatal nurse to know whether a baby is lying in a relaxed way or is just plain tired out. And it may take time to realize that if your baby turns his gaze or his head away when you are looking at his face, talking gently to him or stroking him, this is a positive sign. It is not a rejection of you; it may merely mean that he needs a rest just at this moment, and is mature enough now to be able to break contact in this way – or he may have noticed something interesting over there. A very sick or very immature baby might not be able do this.

Premature babies often drop – alarmingly abruptly – into a sudden light sleep, but that usually just means they have had enough and so they have shut the world out. If your baby does this you might feel he would like to be put back in his cot for a rest, or he might prefer you to hold him quietly, shading his eyes, until he wakes again.

Positive signs

There are many positive signs. For example, when you see your baby showing any of the signs listed above left, it probably means that he is feeling comfortable. If he is doing – or even trying to do – any of the things listed below left it means that he can, or is trying to, comfort himself, without having to wait for you or a nurse to see what is needed and do it for him.

Making it easier

However, if you notice your baby trying to do any of these things listed but not quite making it, you can help him succeed. Perhaps he is taking what look like swipes at his face, but you feel he is really trying to get his fingers into his mouth – you can help by gently bringing his fingers up to his mouth. Are your baby's fingers moving over or scrabbling at his blanket? He may be trying to hold it for comfort – slide a corner into his hand for him to hold.

Signs that your baby might like help

If your baby has scooted down into the corner of his cot he may have done this because he didn't like all that space around him – it may feel very empty after being in the womb. Perhaps he could have some soft nesting (see page 94) around him as boundaries to make him feel secure? He may also need this if he stretches out his legs to touch the sides, but sometimes it may be that he just likes to stretch.

Frowning may just mean he is concentrating, but grimacing or making a face usually means he is not happy about something and would like some help. If his eyes are dull, this may be because his systems are very immature, it

A yawn can be a sign that he needs more oxygen – or he may just be tired.

When your baby

★ has stiff or tense arms, legs or body

★ has a stressed or taut look on his face

★ is being frantically active and cannot seem to calm down

★ has a mottled, paler, dusky or very red skin colour

★ is breathing fast and/or his heartbeat has suddenly speeded up

something is either physically not right or is bothering him

Changes in heartbeat and breathing

It is normal for the heartbeat and breathing rate of premature babies to speed up and slow down, sometimes several times a day. This will stop when their circulatory and nervous systems settle down and mature, unless they have a long-term problem that needs treatment. Your baby's doctors and nurses would soon notice if he did have a problem, and would make sure he had the medical or surgical treatment he needed.

may mean that he is in pain – or it may just be that he wants to go to sleep.

Usually if your baby has a panicky expression in his eyes, with his gaze 'locked' on something, this means that he is having difficulty in coping with whatever is happening to him at the moment, but cannot seem to pull away from it on his own. In this case he may need you to help him by cutting back on anything which is disturbing or stimulating him: perhaps by tucking him up cosily in his cot and shading his eyes, or as far as possible quietening any noise going on nearby, or holding him quietly without rocking or moving. However, some babies also use this 'locked' gaze as a way of calming themselves.

Signs of trouble

In the column on the left are some signs that may suggest that something is physically not right – though, again, it may simply be that your baby is having difficulty coping with whatever is happening to him at the moment. If you see any of these signs, ask a nurse if they could come and check him with you.

OBSERVING AND INTERPRETING YOUR BABY

Even the youngest premature babies are born with their own distinctive personalities, their own likes and dislikes. One may like his feet being lightly held, another may get upset if she is not partially covered up when her nappy is changed, one may be placid, another irritable.

As his parents, you are probably the people who spend most time with your baby. Have you seen how he reacts to having his nappy changed, a blood test taken, his breathing tube suctioned if he is on a ventilator? What helps calm him down when he is upset? What seems to make him comfortable? Have you noticed that anything particular seems to upset him?

Detailed observation like this can give everyone vital information about the best way to handle your baby, so tell your baby's nurses what you have noticed.

PROTECTING YOUR BABY'S SLEEP

Plenty of sleep is very important in helping premature babies grow, especially if they have not been well. Unfortunately they often don't get it because they tend to be disturbed too often. These disturbances include staff carrying out medical procedures, noise, lights that are too bright, alarms going off on equipment, the unit's telephone, even the buzzer on the SCBU door.

There are several things you might like to try to protect your baby from disturbance. You can ask if people could talk very softly when they are near your baby and he is sleeping and put a sign on his cot asking for quiet, to remind them. Find out from the medical staff whether regular interventions, like blood sampling or nappy changing, could be scheduled together as far as is practical, so your baby has chunks of peace and quiet, and

Some parents have found it useful to hang a notice on their baby's cot, to help the medical staff understand him. On it they put details about the baby, such as his name and who his parents are; what he likes (for example, being shaded from bright lights); and what he doesn't like (such as loud voices talking across his cot).

A sheet draped over the top of the incubator shields the baby's eyes from the bright lights of the SCBU.

Tips for keeping your baby undisturbed

★ Turn off any lights near your baby when they are not being used.

★ Ask for a screen to shield your baby if he is near another baby who is receiving phototherapy.

★ Pad any drawer under the incubator, or nearby bin, that keeps banging.

★ If your baby's cot is in earshot of the unit's shrilling telephone or door buzzer, ask to move him somewhere quieter or to turn down the phone's ring to a softer level, or ask whether the phone could be replaced with one that does not ring out loud but instead has an alarm that lights up.

Disturbed rest

Research has shown that, in most neonatal units, babies are disturbed every four to ten minutes.

also whether it is possible for him to have a nap hour in the morning and one in the afternoon when doctors and other caregivers do not disturb him for check-ups and tests unless they are urgent. Some units have a system of quiet periods, often in the afternoon. During these Quiet Times, only parents are can handle and be with their babies, unless there is an emergency. Premature babies ideally need quiet hours during the day *and* night.

PROTECTING YOUR BABY'S EYES

A baby's eyes are the last sensory organs to develop. This means that they are the most immature organs at birth, even for term babies. It makes sense, therefore, to protect premature babies' eyes until they have had a chance to mature. However, SCBUs are usually brightly lit places. Research suggests that, in some cases, the lighting levels are up to a third higher than recommended, and some studies further indicate that this may be associated with damage to premature babies' vulnerable, still-developing eyesight. On the other hand, staff take a risk that, if they cover the incubator to protect against bright light, they could fail to spot problems with the baby or the equipment inside, such as a blockage in a vital tube.

Some American SCBUs use padded incubator covers, because it is thought they help protect premature babies' immature eyes from possible damage from bright lighting, and also help them rest. The padding reduces noise levels too. There are also a few UK units that cover incubators.

Partial covering

Some SCBUs take the middle route, partially covering some of the incubators so the babies' heads are in shade but their bodies and any monitor wires or tubing are still under bright light and so easy to check. This method of partial shading is recommended by some specialists, especially if the baby is medically unstable or critically ill. So if your baby's unit does not cover the incubator you could suggest that a blanket or baby quilt be draped over at least the top half of the cot.

POSITIONING: HOW TO HELP YOUR BABY LIE COMFORTABLY IN THE INCUBATOR

If you look at the way a premature baby lies in his cot, then at the way a newborn term baby lies, you may notice that term babies often lie in a curled-up position, tucked around themselves. But premature babies have weak muscle tone and, if they are not supported in any way and left on their backs, tend to sprawl, legs akimbo and arms flung out sideways. Many parents feel instinctively that it is uncomfortable for their babies to lie like this. There is no specific scientific evidence for that, but it certainly *looks* uncomfortable.

However, there is a growing amount of medical research which suggests that if premature babies are helped and supported to lie in better positions, this can help them develop normal posture and muscle tone. This is important because it means that they will be far more likely to sit, crawl, walk, and move their arms and legs normally as they grow up – these are things which premature babies do tend to have problems with (see page 186–7). Both nurses and parents can help with positioning. This is the practical art of gently supporting premature babies so that they lie in the best and most comfortable positions in their incubators. Positioning helps babies to lie in ways that are likely to be comfortable, but also encourages them to practise gently flexing their muscles, or to push against boundaries. This in turn helps their bodies to develop normally.

Flexion

Babies who have been born too early have not yet had the opportunity to build up enough strength or muscle tone to lie comfortably in a flexed position (curled over), or to support themselves, as a term baby does. The usual way that babies develop some muscle tone is by pushing their arms, legs, hands, feet and shoulders against the womb's walls from time to time – a kind of 'working out' in the womb. Neonatal staff call this flexion. The bigger a baby grows, they less space he has in the womb, the more he flexes against its walls and the more muscle tone he

Movement and posture problems affecting their ability to support their own heads and to sit up unaided are very common in premature babies. In their first year at least 40 per cent – and possibly up to 80 per cent – of premature babies born weighing less than 1,600g (3½lb) are affected. Good positioning can help prevent these problems developing.

Positioning tips

* Place soft supports for his hips, knees, shoulders, neck and side.

* Change his head position regularly.

* Raise the head end of his cot to a 30 degree angle.

* Change the position he lies in from time to time.

* Nest him.

* Place soft boundaries around him to encourage him to flex against them.

* Bring his hands up close to his mouth.

* Put him in the balanced 'midline' position, again bringing his hands up near his mouth.

* Read his body language to check he is comfortable.

* Place him lying on his front; this may help if your baby is finding it difficult to breathe.

develops. This is partly why the earlier a baby is born, the less muscle strength and tone he has.

How to position a baby

You can use soft rolls of flannelette baby sheets, small foam shapes or even mini bean bags to support your baby's small body. These aids also give a baby something to flex against. There are also specially made supports from specialist manufacturers, but these are more expensive. The supports may be placed at all or any of the following places: hips, back, shoulders, knees, or neck.

SCBU staff may also nest a baby by tucking a roll of fabric all the way around the body. This means that he can be supported to lie in the best position for encouraging good posture and muscular development, and to feel comfortably contained and secure as he used to be in the womb. A nest will also give him something to push his feet against, or support his arms so he can bring his hands up to his mouth more easily.

Premature babies are not usually keen on having a lot of space around them and some have repeatedly been found in the corner of their cots if they are strong enough to inch their way down there. If your baby likes to do this, let him be. He will waste more energy trying to find the boundaries he is searching for, if he is constantly being repositioned.

How good positioning can help your baby

Not only can this help develop normal movement and posture, it can also make a baby's breathing easier and encourage a regular heartbeat. Being supported in a more comfortable position can help promote more regular sleeping patterns.

It is also an aid to good digestion: placing a premature baby so he is supported comfortably on his right side can help reduce gastric reflux, a common problem for premature babies (see page 166).

Good positioning helps prevent the unhappy, and sometimes frantic, fidgeting that neonatal staff call 'purposeless movement'. Premature babies can become surprisingly agitated, moving around a good deal when they are distressed or uncomfortable, and this uses up energy and calories that the babies need for growing and recovery. The more comfortable and well supported a baby is, the less he will fidget, the less stressed he is likely to be, and the faster he will gain the weight he needs.

Preventing head flattening

Careful positioning can also avoid 'head flattening'. The development of a slightly misshapen head and face is quite common in babies and toddlers who have been born very early, before 28 weeks. It can happen because the bones of a premature baby's skull are still quite soft, so that when his relatively large head presses down (quite heavily, because he has weak neck muscles) against the surface he lies on, this can press his skull slightly out of shape. The result can be a flattening of the back or sides of the head,

Overheating

If a baby is very premature and finds it especially hard to control his own body temperature, he needs to be checked very regularly to make sure that the nesting materials are not making him too hot.

Gently turning a baby's head at regular intervals can help prevent head flattening.

Front or back at home?

It is completely safe for a baby to sleep on his front in the SCBU, where he is closely monitored all the time. However, when you take your baby home, it is much safer for him to sleep on his back (see pages 171–2). This is why many SCBUs will begin getting babies who have been happily sleeping on their fronts in hospital used to sleeping on their backs before they go home.

and a high narrow forehead and eyes which seem to be placed more to the sides than is usual.

To prevent head flattening, the baby's head needs to be turned regularly, although there is no agreement as yet on exactly how often. Some units do this every two hours, some every six. Some also alternate placing a baby on his back to sleep with placing him on his front. Various aids are also used, though, again, there are no firm conclusions yet about which work best. They include water pillows, water beds, soft air-filled mattresses and soft doughnut-shaped head supports. If you are concerned about head-flattening, ask your baby's medical staff what they recommend to help prevent this.

Front or back?

It also matters whether your baby is laid on his front (prone), back (supine), side or a mixture of all three. Most neonatal units used to nurse sick premature babies on their backs. This was partly so that the staff could see quickly and easily how they were, and partly because it was easier to position SCBU equipment such as umbilical catheters and ventilator tubes. However, over the last few years many research studies have suggested that premature babies used up too much energy, and had lower levels of oxygen in their blood, when they were laid on their backs.

There are major advantages to babies' sleeping on their fronts. These include using up less energy (premature babies have little to spare), spending more time asleep, less fidgeting and restless movement (which again helps save what little energy they have for recovery and growing), a slower heart rate and more stable breathing. There is also evidence that raising the head end of a baby's mattress to a 30 degree angle helps his digestion, lungs and heart to work better.

THERAPEUTIC TOUCH

Despite its name, this is a no-touch method of 'massaging', which uses the natural healing energy from a parent's or nurse's hands held roughly 5–10cm (2–4in) or so away from the baby's body. It is something parents can try on even the very smallest premature baby, and therapeutic touch can often be used for babies who are too fragile or unwell to be massaged, even very lightly, in the usual way.

Therapeutic touch may sound a bit strange and 'New Age', but it is well accepted by many nurses and has been validated by the English National Board of Nursing. It is also being taught to a growing number of British nurses and midwives. Its benefits are backed up by dozens of clinical research trials, though only one or two have been carried out specifically on premature babies in SCBUs. In America, more than 80 universities both use and teach the therapy. According to clinical trials, the technique appears to have a deep relaxing effect, can reduce pain, soothe anxiety and distress, and may also help wounds and injuries heal faster.

You could ask a nurse trained in this type of no-touch massage to do it for your baby (see *Helplines*, page 200. But you can also easily learn how to do it yourself. As the mother or father of your baby, you are an especially good person to do this because you love your child so much, and know him better than anyone else.

Some parents find they prefer a bit of temporary privacy when they use therapeutic touch for their baby, and ask if they might have some screens around them for a little while.

CONTAINMENT CARE

This is another kind of treatment you might like to try, if your baby is not ready for even the gentlest massage just yet. With containment care you cup your hand around your baby's head, without quite touching it. Leave your hand in position, and imagine warmth and energy flowing from your hand into his head.

You can take this further when you feel your baby is ready (check with your baby's nurses or doctors): cup your hand around his head just touching it, gently cradling his feet with your other hand.

Even the tiniest premature babies usually like this. This may be because it gives them a sense of being safely held in a limited space, as they were in the womb.

Therapeutic touch by parents

1 Sit down by your baby, preferably at a time when he is fairly settled, not due to be handled, for example for nappy changing or any medical tests, and not hungry, and the SCBU is fairly quiet. Look at him and focus all your attention on him. Try – as one nurse trained in therapeutic touch put it – to 'send him your love, with your eyes'. Do this for a few moments – as long as feels right to you.

2 Now hold one of your hands, palms down, about 5–10cm (2–4in) above your baby's head, and the other a similar distance from his feet. You could use your fingers for this instead if you feel that your palms are 'too big' for your tiny baby. Try to send him your love through your hands or fingers.

3 If you would like to do a little more, try slowly 'stroking' your baby from his head to his feet, again keeping your hands 5–10cm (2–4in) away from his body. Do this for as much time as you feel is right. Most parents spend only a minute or two.

4 To finish, bring your hands or fingers back to their original position, just above your baby's head and feet, let them stay there for a few seconds, then end.

97

COMFORT AND CONTACT

Almost all parents of even the tiniest or most fragile of premature babies have a powerful instinct to stroke, lay their hands upon, and soothe their own infants. Mothers or fathers will get to know instinctively just the sort of contact their baby needs, or can cope with. There are many things parents can do to make contact with their premature babies, even when they are too fragile or unwell to be picked up and cuddled.

Talking to your baby

Talking to your baby gently and quietly is a very natural thing for any parent to do, and is an excellent and effective way of making contact with your baby, no matter how young he is. If he shows any signs – such as yawning or turning his head – that he is finding this attention too much to cope with, leave it for a bit and try again later, using your baby's responses as your guide.

Placing your index finger gently in his hand

Even extremely premature babies can grasp with their hands (although strong grasp reflexes do not come until a baby is 32 weeks or more, and actual muscle tone tends to develop relatively late, from 34–36 weeks) and they find it comforting to have something to hold on to. In the womb from about 24 weeks their hands are big enough to grasp their umbilical cord; pictures of babies this age captured on ultrasound often show them doing so. Some researchers have suggested that this is a baby's first comforter, and that even when he is still in the peace of the womb, it helps him feel more secure. Holding your finger may bring that feeling back, as well as giving him precious physical contact with you.

Letting him suck the tip of your little finger

Babies of all ages find sucking very soothing. Your baby will have been practising sucking movements since he was only 1l–12 weeks old in your womb, and a few weeks after that he may have co-ordinated his thumb into his mouth, as many ultrasound scan pictures show. If you find that your baby likes to suckle on your little finger, make sure

Holding him close

10 baby-comforting ideas

★ Reduce any stress from his surroundings (for example, from noise or bright light).

★ Make sure he is lying supported in a comfortable position in his cot.

★ Put your hands gently on his bottom or back if he is frantic or restless.

★ Cup one hand gently around his head, the other gently touching his feet.

★ Swaddle him (with his arms free) and lay him on his side in his incubator with some kind of cover shading his eyes.

★ Hold him close without rocking or talking.

★ Speak softly to him without making eye contact.

★ 'Think' calm, love and energy into him.

★ Give him your little finger to suck or hold.

★ Wrap him in a blanket and hold him quietly.

★ Place him comfortably within a cosy 'nest' of soft rolls of bedding (check that he doesn't get too hot).

the nail is very short with no sharp edges anywhere, and that both nails and hands are very clean.

However, being able to suck on your finger does not necessarily mean he is ready to breast- or bottle-feed yet. To do this he needs to be able to co-ordinate his sucking, breathing and swallowing.

Gently bringing his hands near his mouth

This encourages him to suck his own fingers and thumbs. Finger and thumb sucking is a really important part of his learning to comfort and calm *himself*, rather than having to wait for you or a nurse to do the comforting for him. Now he is outside the womb, your baby might not yet be able to co-ordinate his movements accurately enough to bring his fingers to his mouth, but it is a good thing if he is trying.

Comforting your baby during interventions

'Interventions' is a catch-all term for anything that involves touching your baby. This could range from a cuddle or a massage to having an IV line or a feeding tube inserted.

As SCBUs have become more high-tech, the number of times premature babies are handled in an average day has increased dramatically. The hospital staff have to do these things to care for your baby and to check on his well-being. Unfortunately, many necessary interventions are thoroughly uncomfortable. Some hurt. And all of them may be disturbing for your baby.

You can lessen the impact of the unpleasant interventions by comforting your baby as they happen, helping to re-settle them afterwards. Parents usually have far more time to do this than nurses do, and because you know your own baby best you will be able to soothe him better than anyone.

Some parents like to be there to support their baby through interventions and to help him settle afterwards. Others find that they can become upset themselves when they see their baby distressed. If this is the case for you, would you perhaps be able to help your baby most by not being there during the procedure itself, but coming to comfort and soothe him immediately afterwards instead?

You may find that whether or not you stay with your baby throughout depends on how you yourself are feeling, how tired you are, how well or unwell your baby is, and on what sort of intervention is being carried out. Follow your feelings and your own instincts. Just do whatever feels right to you at each particular time.

You can comfort your baby by talking to him for a minute or two before the intervention happens. Some parents find they like to talk to their baby as if he were a much older child. They explain quietly what will happen, and that it won't last long. Your baby may well catch your drift and appreciate it, even though he will not understand your actual words.

During the intervention you could give your baby your finger to hold or suckle on, cup a hand around his head, put a reassuring hand against his back, or gently touch his arm or hand. Afterwards it is important to soothe him until he is calm and relaxed again. Premature babies have not yet developed the skills they need to calm themselves back down after being upset. They are what SCBU staff call 'disorganized', meaning that their nervous systems are not yet developed enough for them to return quickly to normal after something has upset or disturbed them. They need your help to do this.

HOLDING YOUR BABY

You can hold even the tiniest of premature babies from 24 or 25 weeks, so long as they are medically stable – that is: though they may be ill, they are holding steady and not getting any worse. If you want to hold your own baby for a little while, it is your right to do so. Do not take no for an answer if staff seem reluctant, unless there is a good medical reason why your child must not be disturbed at all for the moment. Talk to your baby's paediatrician or neonatologist about this if you are not sure whether your baby is medically stable or not, or if you are still not being encouraged to hold him.

'At first I used to feel stupid, leaning over a 33-week-old premature baby and saying something like "Look sweetheart, Mum's really sorry but you have to have this blood test done now. I know it isn't very nice but it will only be for a moment … there, it's OK now…" just as you would for an older baby or toddler. But then I thought: who's to say an older baby understands you word for word, but that doesn't stop most parents chatting away to them, does it?'

Valerie, Lee's mother

'I was grateful to all the nurses, I really was. They were being so kind to us, and they had saved Gail's life. But when I saw them doing all these things for her, even kissing her head and stroking her back to soothe her – I felt sick with jealousy, and anger. That was my baby. How dare those other women stroke the top of her head like that? Then tell me she was still too fragile to be picked up by me, her mother?'

Jo, mother of Gail, born at 31 weeks

'I was looking forward to holding Scarlett in my arms so much after she had been in an incubator and on a ventilator. But when it came down to it and they gave her to me, I sat there rigid with nerves. I was so afraid of pulling out a vital tube or line from her life-support system that I didn't dare move. It was only for 10 minutes but it seemed a lot longer because I was so worried and nervous. I remember how relieved I was to give her back again. Then I felt upset, and guilty for not enjoying it more ... yet a few weeks later I was picking her up very confidently, wires and all, as if I was a nurse.'

Ashleigh, mother of Scarlett,
who was born at 32 weeks

'Kangaroo care is simply the best you can do to help your premature infant. And it is a procedure that does not cost a penny ...'

Dr Susan Ludington-Hoe, US
kangaroo care pioneer and
researcher at UCLA School
of Nursing

Tiny and frail though he is, John is comfortable and safe in his mother's arms, and with his sister's gentle touch.

When they're all wired up . . .

Many parents have said that though they wanted very much to hold their babies properly, they found it quite alarming the first couple of times.

Don't worry if a tube comes out while you are holding or picking up your baby – that's always happening. Some neonatal nurses say that it often seems as if one of premature babies' favourite occupations is pulling their tubes out by themselves. There is no need to panic as it is really not much of a problem, nor is it a bar to lifting your baby out yourself. Just call a nurse and she will put the tube back in again.

KANGAROO CARE

Kangaroo care is a way of holding your premature baby so that she rests on your chest, with her bare skin against yours. It can be very good – from a medical point of view – for the babies themselves. It can be good for parents too because it feels close and loving: it means you can have some real physical contact with your baby and it offers a gentle, hands-on way of really mothering or fathering your own child.

Babies can be held this way even when they are very small and premature. The most important factors affecting whether your baby can have kangaroo care are whether: your baby is medically stable (see page 106); the SCBU nurses are familiar with this way of holding a premature baby; and the medical staff are confident about supporting you in doing this.

Those SCBUs that can help you give your baby kangaroo care will normally be happy for this to begin at around 30 weeks. Some units have staff who are very practised and confident in this area, and are happy to begin even earlier: neonatal staff who are experienced in encouraging kangaroo care say that you can safely 'kangaroo' a baby as tiny as 600g (1 lb 6oz).

If your baby is very premature or very small he is probably being monitored and tube-fed, and he may have CPAP (see page 30) too. This means he will be attached to some lead wires and tubes, so you will have to sit or recline

near the equipment and not move around much. If your baby is older or more mature and does not need close monitoring, you can move around carefully, holding him tucked down your front. Many parents like to lie back on a sofa, a bed in one of the parents' rooms, or in an armchair or rocking chair with their feet up.

How kangaroo care helps your baby

One question many parents ask about kangaroo care is how something so simple, natural and low-tech can make such a difference to the health of a premature baby. There are several good medical reasons why, but perhaps the simple answer is that babies like it. They are comfortable in the warmth, closeness, peace and security of being held close to their mother or father. Perhaps it reminds them of the safety of the womb they left too early.

What is clear is that their health improves tremendously. There has been an immense amount of international research backing up the benefits of kangaroo care, from the UK, the US, Scandinavia, Germany and France, to India and Central and South America. UNICEF and The World Health Organization also recommend it.

Premature babies sleep better and breathe more easily when they are being 'kangaroo'd'. They cry and fidget less and, being calmer, they grow better. If babies have regular kangaroo care, they also breast-feed more easily, and their mothers can keep making milk for longer.

Kangaroo'd babies have fewer apnoea (stop-breathing) and bradycardia (slowed heartbeat) attacks, and fewer body-temperature fluctuations – they stay warm, thanks to the warmth of your body. They develop fewer infections, leave their incubators sooner, and go home earlier.

Benefits for parents

Kangaroo care can be immensely comforting and calming for parents. Touching skin-to-skin and relaxing, without the artificial barriers of special care cot and any medical equipment, it is easier for you to bond with your baby.

How to give kangaroo care

Wear something that unbuttons down the front, and wash your hands, to cut down the possibility of infection.

1 It is a good idea to put a cotton bonnet on your baby if he is not already wearing one – babies lose a lot of heat from their heads; but take off the rest of his clothes, or at least undo them at the front.

2 Undo the front of your clothes, lift your baby from his incubator and lay him on his tummy between your breasts (fathers should lay their baby on their chests).

3 Your baby's position is very important: so that he can breathe easily, he needs to lie on his tummy and upright against you, with his head turned to one side; make sure he is not slumped, or curled up. Ask the nurses to help you if you would like some support.

4 Tuck him inside your clothes and hold him there, as if he were a baby kangaroo in a mother kangaroo's pouch.

The best position for you to be in while holding him like this, especially at first, is sitting down and leaning slightly back, perhaps with your feet up, so that he rests easily on you. You could perhaps put a blanket around him, over your clothes, to help hold him in place.

Held in skin-to-skin contact with her mother, as close as she can possibly be, Gabrielle is comfortable and content.

Ready for massage

Generally, a premature baby can be gently massaged on his back if he:

★ Is medically stable (see below). This is very important, because any touch for a premature baby who is still medically unstable can be distressing for him.

★ Is at least 28 weeks corrected age (see page 157), *or* four to six weeks old.

★ Is able to cope with having his nappy changed by his mother and father.

★ Is able to keep his own temperature fairly steady.

★ Has no lines or tubes which prevent him from being turned over on his stomach.

★ Does not need tube-feeding (see page 113).

You may even be able to massage your baby if he is on a ventilator because he has a long-term condition, such as BPD, but is otherwise medically stable.

medically stable means still ill but holding steady and not getting any worse.

MASSAGE

Massaging can be a gentle way to show your love and care for your premature baby, and to soothe and comfort him. It also has proven health benefits, and many SCBUs encourage mothers and fathers to massage their premature babies if the infants can cope with it. Research suggests it can have many positive effects, including improving digestion, helping babies sleep more soundly and deeply, encouraging them to breathe more easily, raising the levels of oxygen in their bloodstream, steadying their heart rate and even helping them gain weight more quickly.

Is your baby ready to be massaged?

Premature babies can be highly sensitive to touch. The more premature or unwell they are, the more hyper-sensitive they tend to be. Because of this, your baby may not be able to cope with a massage just yet. In some cases, unless the unit's neonatal nurses are trained in massaging premature babies, it may not be possible to give your child his first 'proper' massage until he is nearly ready to go home. A very little gentle stroking or holding may be suggested instead.

When your baby has a small massage, you should not see his need for oxygen increase any more than it would when you change his nappy. After the massage, his level of oxygen saturation (the amount of oxygen in his blood) should go back to 'resting level' or even increase slightly. If his oxygen saturation level drops or goes up sharply, this is a sign of stress, and would suggest that he is not able to cope with a massage yet. SCBU staff may also advise that you do not give your baby a massage if he is having a bit of an 'off' day – perhaps is having more spells of apnoea or bradycardia than is normal for him, is seeming more lethargic than usual, or has been handled a lot that day already for tests or x-rays.

Every baby is highly individual. If you are not too sure about whether your baby is ready for a brief, light massage, talk about it to the nurse who knows him best, or the paediatrician or neonatologist. Keep a close eye on your baby's signals (see page 86) and use your own instincts as a parent to check that he is coping each time you give him even a small massage. If you are not sure whether he is ready just yet, perhaps it might be better to try some therapeutic touch or containment care (see page 97) to soothe him, until he is stronger and his nervous system is more mature.

How to massage your premature baby

There are different schools of thought about the 'best' way to massage a premature baby. You may be in a SCBU which has its own particular way of massaging, which they could teach you and help you with. However, for most parents, a formula approach is not really what massaging their baby is about, and it is not the massage technique itself that is important. What matters most is your finding a safe way of enjoying loving contact with your baby.

Try to do your baby's massage at roughly the same time each day, and pick a quiet time. A good time is when there are no daily ward rounds going on, he is not hungry and he has not had anything done to him which may have upset and tired him (such as a blood test, tube suctions, a nappy change or a wash). Get everything ready first: some cotton wool, a little oil in a container standing in warm water and perhaps some music he likes (anything you know he can relax with).

Use plain vegetable oil. *Never* use aromatherapy oils on a premature baby's skin: they are too strong even when diluted down by a carrier oil. Do not use commercial baby oils, either, as they are mineral-based.

During the massage, always leave part of one hand or a fingertip on your baby, so that you never completely stop touching him. If you want to cover part of him up a little more, or dip the cotton wool into a bit more warm oil, keep, say, the back of one of your hands in contact with him as you do so.

How often you can massage depends on how well, or how fragile, your baby is at the moment. Many parents say they began with two or three times a week, working up to once a day if their baby liked it and could cope with this. Neonatal staff advise not mixing kangaroo care, cuddles

A gentle massage for a premature baby

1 Undo your baby's clothing to waist level.

2 Dab some cotton wool in the oil and gently smooth a little on your baby's back.

3 Place your hands over your baby's back, but not touching him. Pause so he gets used to your hands being there.

4 Gently massage his back with your right hand, your left hand lying gently on the back of his neck. Using just two fingertips, massage in small circles down by one side of your baby's spine (without touching the spine itself) and back up the other side.

5 Repeat using bigger circles (with more oil if needed).

6 Make the circles bigger still, going from the baby's back around to his abdomen.

7 To end, wipe off the excess oil with cotton wool, stroke his back gently, then pause for a moment with your hands just above his back.

8 Cover him gently with a blanket for the moment, rather than disturbing him by dressing him again.

After a massage

Afterwards, it is a good idea to hang a notice on the end of his cot, saying something like: *'Just had a massage. Please do not disturb.'* Write the time at the end of it, so the nurses know how long to leave him resting.

and a massage all in the same day unless you can see from your baby's signals that he can definitely manage all this.

If there is a nurse at your SCBU who knows about premature baby massage, you may like to get her to show you the first time, do the massage with her the second, and do it by yourself the third time, with her watching or helping. If not, you could ask the nurse who knows your baby best if she could support and help you to try the simple massage on page 107, and see if your baby likes it.

Premature baby massage guidelines are there to help parents find out and learn about ways of touching their baby which are enjoyable (for both parties) and safe. It is very important to watch your baby's reactions: be guided by them, more than anything else. Is there anything special he seems to like? Or not like? Does he seem relaxed when you massage him? How does your baby let you know when he has had enough?

Back to sleep

It is fine to leave your baby sleeping on his front after a massage when he is in the SCBU and attached to monitors which can tell you whether he is breathing well or not, and whether his heart rate is regular. At home, however, it is safest to turn your baby gently on to his back after 15 minutes or so, before you let him carry on sleeping.

If your baby cries

Try not to feel too discouraged if your baby cries the first time he has a massage, or even the second or third time too. This may be because most of the touching he has had up until now has not been very pleasant. In fact, most of his experience of touch may have been uncomfortable or even painful. If a baby is usually only touched for nappy changing, blood sampling from his heel, being medically examined, having his IV lines or feeding tubes changed, it is not surprising that he may associate touch with something bad happening to him. But if you massage your baby regularly, he will come to associate your type of gentle touching or massage with pleasure and reassurance instead.

PLAYING WITH YOUR PREMATURE BABY

This may not be 'playing' in the sense you use with an older baby. However, it *is* play, if play is defined as something that catches and holds your baby's interest, *and which he can join in with.* Your premature baby may be able to cope with a little of this type of interaction at around 33 or 34 weeks. But how much he will be able to manage depends on many different things, including how well or unwell he is, what medical problems he has had, and how he has been cared for. It also depends upon whether or not your baby has any particular medical condition which means he might find this sort of interaction especially tiring or hard to deal with.

You will not necessarily need bright rattles, or soft cuddly toys, though you might like to try showing them to your baby, perhaps just placing them in his cot, to see if he is interested. Try to put a toy like this within his sight line but so he can easily move his gaze away if he does not want to look at it. However, he will probably be more interested in your face, touch and voice.

How long to play

The awake time for a premature baby aged 33–34 weeks can vary greatly depending on many different factors – the same ones that determine how ready he is for play. However, even if he is well and has been cared for very sensitively and protectively, you will probably find that he can only cope with very brief period of interaction or concentration: perhaps a couple of minutes at the most. This may not sound like much. Yet if you think that if your baby had not been born early he would never have felt the touch of a hand, or even looked at anything, for several weeks yet, it may begin to seem like a good deal.

So long as your baby is well and stable, a good time to try interacting with him is when he is rested, calm and awake of his own accord – that is, has not been woken up by someone else. Find out if there are any regular times when your baby is awake and time playtime for one of these. If there are no regular times yet, just sit quietly by

Playing with your premature baby

SCBU nursing staff suggest that there are three important things to remember:

1 Find the right time.

2 Only do one thing at a time.

3 Be guided by your baby's own signals (see page 86).

your baby (perhaps reading or trying to rest) until he is awake and seems alert.

At 34 weeks premature babies can usually only cope with one thing at a time. Your baby may enjoy touch, listening, and looking. But dealing with all three (or even two) forms of stimulation at once is usually too much.

Try to observe your baby while you are 'playing' with him. He is telling you how he feels with his body language, the expression on his face, the way he is holding his hands or arms, his muscle tension, the rate of his breathing and his heart rate, even the colour tone of his skin. Does he seem to you to be coping with the contact, and enjoying it? Or do you feel that perhaps now is not such a good time? Be guided by your baby's signals and try to trust your own instincts as a parent too – they are usually right.

Touching

Try holding or stroking softly along his hand, foot or back. If your baby can cope with this, try feeling his arms and legs, gently but not with a feathery-light touch – babies do not seem to like that. If he does not seem comfortable with this, leave it and try again another time. There may be other forms of touching that your own baby especially likes. Some premature babies find a hand cupping the head soothing. Others like their feet being held, or their shoulders supported by an adult's hand. If your baby is well enough for a bath, you may well find that he loves being held securely in the gently moving water.

Looking

Let your baby see your face about 20–25cm (8–10in) away. Smile or just look at him calmly and 'speak' with your eyes. Allow him to focus on your face. Then slowly move your head from side to side. Watch to see if his eyes follow you. You may notice that even about half a minute of this may be enough. If your baby seems ready and interested in interacting with you in this way, even for short periods, the play-looking can help him to develop and co-ordinate his sight.

Talking

Talk softly to your baby, recite nursery rhymes, poetry – anything you feel comfortable saying to him and that you feel he might like to listen to. If you begin to see signals that you know mean your baby would prefer just to be peaceful for now without any stimulation, leave it for a while and try again later.

FEEDING YOUR PREMATURE BABY

Feeding a premature baby can at first look like a difficult and specialized job that only the nurses can do, especially if the baby is very premature, fragile or unwell. But it isn't.

If you would like to be properly involved in feeding your own baby and have enough time to do it, you can. In fact, you are probably the best person in the world to do it. Some units are 100 per cent behind parents who want to

Even though he needs a nasal cannula to help him breathe, he can still enjoy being bathed by his mother.

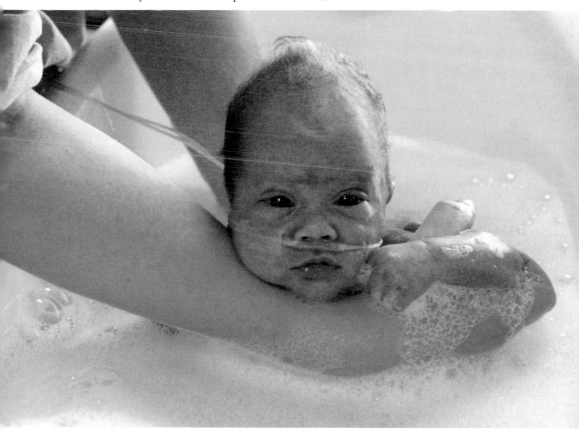

A premature baby's food will contain:

★ more calories for energy, as a premature baby can use up a great deal, especially if he is stressed or unwell

★ more fat, since he needs this for energy but will not have much of his own stored up yet

★ more protein, which is very important for growing

★ more water, because premature babies can become dehydrated very quickly and their water intake needs to be carefully and individually monitored

★ more vitamins and minerals, because a baby usually builds up his stores in the last 12 weeks he spends in his mother's womb; the earlier your baby was born, the lower his store of vital minerals and vitamins will be

feed their own babies, others are less enthusiastic. However, with the staff's support, parents can help with all the different premature baby feeding methods, including tube-feeds.

Either the mother or father (or both) can take over the responsibility for tube-feeding, bottle-feeding, cup-feeding and (if you are the mother) eventually breast-feeding your baby. Depending on how much time you can spend at the SCBU, you can do this part-time, so that a certain feed time or times are saved for you when you can come into the unit, or almost full-time, if you are able to be around most of the time, just going home for a few hours each night to get some sleep.

Mothers can also do something else very special for their babies that no one else can – give them their expressed breast-milk. This is probably the single most important thing you can do to help your baby grow strong and well. Even if you only make a little bit, this will still be very valuable for your baby, and it can be topped up with formula. However, if you find you cannot express your milk, you can still be fully involved in your own baby's care by using a tube, cup or bottle to give them a special premature-formula baby milk instead.

What babies need

Premature babies want feeding and nourishing just like other babies. It is just that they need to be fed in different ways until they are able to co-ordinate their sucking, swallowing and breathing to take their milk from the breast, or from a bottle, for themselves. (They can often suck on your finger or a dummy quite strongly long before they can breast- or bottle-feed.) They also need a special milk mixture until their digestive systems and kidneys reach the 'term baby' stage.

IV feeding

IV (intravenous) feeding involves giving special liquid feed via a fine tube, into a vein. At first the liquid feed will be a mixture of sugar (glucose), salts and water; later some amino acids (protein building blocks), plus some fats and minerals may be added. IV feeding is used when a baby is too premature (from 23 to 28 weeks), too small (under 1,000g/2lb 3oz) or too unwell to digest milk. It may be given for the first few hours or even first few days after birth, depending on how prematurely the baby was born and also on how well or unwell he is.

So long as the baby is well and stable enough, even while he is being fed intravenously he may also be able to cope with beginning to learn to enjoy licking milk from his mother's nipple as a preliminary to breast-feeding.

Tube-feeding

This method feeds milk through a fine plastic tube, and is used when your baby's digestive system is ready for feeds by mouth but he cannot yet suckle and drink properly, for himself. The tube usually threads down via the baby's nose or mouth, then into his stomach and is known as a naso-

Ella needs to be fed through a naso-gastric tube, but, touching her own face with one hand and holding tight to her mother's finger with the other, she is serene and relaxed.

Methods of tube-feeding

At the very beginning, the milk may be dripped gently down the tube all the time. This is called *continuous feeding*.

The next stage is hourly feeds, then two-hourly, then every three hours, as your baby is gradually able to cope with larger and larger amounts of milk at a time. This sort of small, regular meal of milk is called a *bolus*.

or oro-gastric tube. There is also another sort of feeding tube which goes straight through the stomach and down into the small intestine. This is called a transpyloric tube. It gives small amounts of milk continuously, and might be used if a baby is very small. Your baby's feed may be formula milk, breast-milk or a mixture of both.

Your baby may be fed by tube alone for several days, for a few weeks or even for a few months – just how long depends on how well he is, and how prematurely he was born. As he becomes more mature and stronger, he can be introduced to cup-feeding, breast-feeding or bottle-feeding gradually, while still having top-up feeds by tube.

You can give your baby small amounts of your breast-milk down this tube right from the very beginning. It is also possible to introduce him to the idea of breast-feeding while he is still tube-feeding, just as soon as he can lick milk off your nipple.

Many units will encourage a mother to hold her baby against her partly bared breast just before a tube-feed when the baby is becoming hungry, then to express a little milk on to her nipple and areola, and position her baby's face so that he can both smell the milk and reach the nipple. If a baby is ready he will often begin to try to lick the milk off. The lovely smell and taste of it, plus the special scent of the mother's skin, can all set the scene to help him begin to try some practice sucking, as a first important step towards learning to breast-feed.

Practice sucking

If your baby is able to do a little practice sucking every time he has a tube-feed, this is very good for him. Research suggests it helps babies' digestion, so they tend to put on weight faster, and helps co-ordinate their breathing-sucking-swallowing, so they can go on to cup-feeding or breast-feeding more quickly. It is best if he can practise suckling on your nipple, but many units also use a dummy.

Positioning your baby in the right way for practice sucking at your breast is very important, and a tiny shift of position can make a huge difference to whether your baby is able to try suckling or not. Hold a baby in one way and it all seems perfectly easy, hold him slightly differently and he is not happy or comfortable so he either won't try, or won't be able to and will get discouraged very quickly.

Try asking the staff to help you if you are not too sure, as many times as you feel you need, since most will be only too glad to support you. If your baby still has a nose tube taped in place, try to hold him so that the tube-free nostril is facing away from your nipple so he can breathe; if he has a tube passing down into his mouth, make sure that it is taped at the side of his mouth and cheek rather than down over his bottom lip and chin.

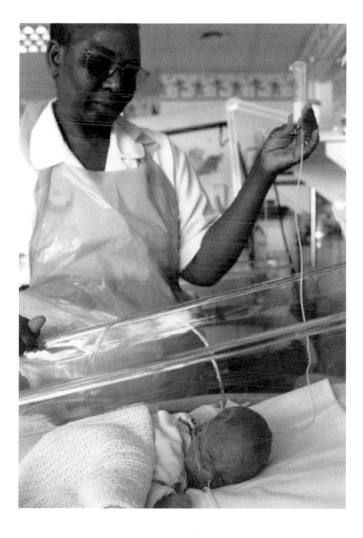

Archie's nurse is feeding him through a naso-gastric tube.

'I couldn't wait for the day when I could first hold Annie on my lap and cup-feed her myself. But I was so scared of pulling out a monitor wire or a tube that when the nurse put her in my arms and encouraged me to feed her I just sat there rigid. It was a relief to put her back and I was so upset I cried buckets afterwards. Yet three weeks later I hardly noticed all the wires and was getting her in and out to feed her all the time on my own, just like a nurse would.'

Jo, Annie's mother

Cup-feeding and breast-feeding

Babies who cup-feed are more likely to be able to breast-feed than babies who don't. As soon as your baby is old enough to lick from a cup he can also lick from you, and you can begin to help him get used to the fact that your breast means food and comfort. This is the beginning of being able to breast-feed.

1 Try to get your baby to lick a little expressed milk off your nipple.

2 When he has got used to this, try expressing a little into his mouth as he nuzzles at your breast.

3 The final stage is helping him latch on to your breast with his mouth so he can try to suckle for himself.

Cup-feeding

With cup-feeding, you hold your baby cuddled comfortably upright on your lap, and gently lift a small cup of milk (like a little medicine cup with rounded edges) to his mouth, tilting it very slightly so a tiny bit goes against his lips. The fact that the milk is against his lips rather than poured into his mouth means that the baby himself is in control of his own drinking, and that he is less likely to choke or become stressed by the fear of choking. Some nurses also suggest swaddling the baby so that he cannot knock the cup with his hands.

Your baby will be able to smell and taste the milk, which he cannot do when he is tube-fed, and because it smells and tastes good this encourages him to try to drink for himself. Within a few days or a week or so he will cotton on to the idea and first begin to lick from the cup, then lap at it like a kitten. Later, he will progress to sipping the milk. The next step is to give him a bottle or try breast-feeding, if you would like to.

Many mothers like to hold their baby against their naked skin, perhaps partly undoing their blouse or lifting their T-shirt, so he can smell its special scent, especially if they are feeding their baby their own breast-milk, and/or planning to try and breast-feed fully later on. Skin-to-skin contact like this or kangaroo care (see page 102) helps your body to make breast-milk too.

A premature baby will probably need a combination of tube-feeding and cup-feeding for several weeks, gradually learning to take more milk from the cup each time, then perhaps having one whole feed from a cup, then two . . . and so on until he takes most or all of his milk like this. (You can continue until your baby is ready to take all his feeds either by breast-feeding or bottle-feeding.) You need not worry about how much milk he drinks this way at first. His nurse will be able to work out if he needs a top up by tube, and if so, how much extra he needs each time.

If your SCBU does not cup-feed their babies If you are interested in feeding your baby this way but the unit does not yet offer it, one possible gentle way into a discussion with your babies' nurses might be to mention that you have been reading something about cup-feeding (perhaps even show them this small section here). Say that you have heard it can triple the rate of successful breast-feeding, which it can. Ask them what their own thoughts are on this. If they seem interested, ask if they might possibly like to talk to staff on a unit that does cup-feed about helping you to do this. Some top SCBUs which use cup-feeding very successfully are listed on page 200. The senior staff there would probably be very glad to talk to nurses from your unit – as one professional to another – about their own experience of it. There is also a book about cup-feeding aimed at nursing professionals which they might find interesting (see *References*).

Bottle-feeding

Once a premature baby is mature enough to manage sucking, swallowing and breathing at the same time, you can begin to feed him using a specially small bottle, which only holds 25–50ml (1–2oz) milk, and a special teat that is as small, soft and flexible as possible. There are many different designs and you may find your baby likes one sort better than another.

The bottle will contain a powdered milk formula mixture that is specially designed for preterm babies. Because his digestive system and organs such as the kidneys and the liver are not mature yet, and because he may be unwell, a premature baby will need a very particular formula mixture customized just for him. Your baby's personal milk mixture may need to be changed and adapted as he grows and matures, and the dietician, paediatrician or neonatologist will follow your baby's progress carefully to suggest changes in the formula mix as and when needed.

Bottle-feeding will help your baby flourish and grow, and you may find that it is the best way for you and your child. Many mothers of premature babies – even those who have successfully breast-fed their other children – find that they cannot breast-feed. This may be because they are often very tired, stressed, not well, have not had the

'One reason given to parents for not cup-feeding is that it could be dangerous because a baby might breathe in the milk. However, this simply isn't true. I think if there had been a single case of this happening in the UK I would have heard about it.'

Sandra Lang, cup-feeding pioneer and Infant Feeding Consultant to the World Health Organization and UNICEF

'I really did try, I stuck at it for eight days. It seemed like forever and I could hardly get any milk out. It was really winding me up. I couldn't believe something so natural was so difficult, and I felt miserable and stupid because it was like – my body couldn't stay pregnant for long enough and now even my boobs didn't work ... So he was fed on formula and he's fine. Getting bigger every day. '

Cherie, Cole's mother

Try to feed him when he's not tired

Does your baby seem to be tired out by having his nappy changed, being dressed, examined by the doctors, having his heel prick tests? If so, try to feed him before any of this is done, or some time afterwards, so he has a chance to recover. Check when any routine tests or procedures will be done and ask the nurses to help you work out a feeding plan timed to avoid these interventions. Suckling takes energy and if he is tired, he will not be able to feed very well.

Enjoying a bottle-feed, and an opportunity for closeness

support needed to breast-feed or simply cannot make enough milk for their premature baby's needs. Some mothers may have other heavy commitments such as a home and other children to care for, have had to return to work, or live a long way away from the unit which mean they are not able to spend very long at the SCBU each day.

Gently preparing your baby In their early weeks of life, it's possible that most of the things happening to a sick, premature baby in or around his mouth have been unpleasant, maybe even painful – endotracheal tubes, feeding tubes, nasal tubes taped and re-taped to his cheeks. Yet you can make sure you offer some gentle touches around your baby's mouth, to help show him that touches in and around his mouth can feel good too. For instance, research suggests that gentle, loving stroking of your baby's lips and around his mouth can make for easier feeding. Offering your baby chances for comfort-sucking can also help. Signs that your baby might like to comfort-suck include trying to bring his hands up to his mouth, turning his head and opening his mouth, and making little sucking movements.

Positioning your baby so both of you are comfortable Hold him with his head slightly raised, close to the warmth of your body, perhaps with his head and upper body against a bared patch of your skin so he can smell and feel you. Ask the nurses to help you here if you are not sure if the position is quite right. A bit of privacy can help create a small oasis of peace and quiet for you both to enjoy the cuddling, closeness, and one-to-one time of the bottle-feed, so if the SCBU is busy, you could ask for screens to be placed around you for a while.

Taking it at your baby's own pace Try to take your time, and let your baby set the pace of the feed. You don't need to hurry it along by wiggling the nipple in your baby's mouth or prodding him gently awake to encourage him to take more or drink a little faster. If he stops suckling, let him rest for a while.

Bottle-feeding can sometimes be a little trickier than breast- or cup-feeding because the milk can flow faster.

'I had always wanted to feed him myself, I had decided right back when I was only a few weeks pregnant I would breast-feed my baby. But I had an emergency caesarean at 29 weeks, and he was so ill at first. I felt bad for several days afterwards, then I was too upset about Michael being in intensive care to really get any expressing going. I just couldn't face it, on top of everything else.'

Kate, Michael's mother

If you would like to breast-feed your premature baby, it is usually better, if possible, not to bottle-feed at all. This is because babies suckle on bottle teats in one way and nipples in another. Trying to learn both at once may confuse your baby, and he may not be able to breast-feed after all. Instead, cup-feeding can be a good halfway house between tube-feeding and breast-feeding.

Prodding the baby, or moving the bottle about, twisting/turning it to get him to take more milk may look like an effective way to get your baby to take in more food and certainly, in the old days, neonatal units took quite a lot of pride in using these methods to make sure babies drank the 'required' amount of milk every time. But most now know that forcing milk down, without the baby drinking it himself, can make feeding stressful for a baby and may cause apnoea and bradycardia attacks.

Try not to be discouraged if, initially, it seems that the nurses can get your baby to feed more than you can. This often happens, perhaps because parents cuddle their baby so gently and lovingly, that, feeling safe and secure, he responds by falling happily asleep. Sitting a baby up and gently winding him can wake him up a little. So can touching the soles of his feet, making eye contact with him or talking to him. However, it may be that what your baby is saying is that he is just not ready at that point to take a whole bottle, but he is ready for a cuddle.

Most units usually suggest 20–30 minutes for a feed, depending on the baby, so as not to tire him right out. If a feed goes on for more than half an hour, it can leave a baby exhausted. Be guided by your own baby's signals – those, and your own special instincts as parents, will let you know better than anything else whether he would like to carry on feeding or stop for now.

Can I breast-feed as well? Mothers' own milk supply usually drops slowly over time if they do bottle-feed. This is because the more stimulation your breasts have, either from a baby's suckling or from expressing, the more milk you will make. The reverse is also true: the less expressing or suckling they receive, the less milk you make.

Breast-feeding

Breast-milk can do many things for your baby that formula milk cannot. It is not just a food – it is a powerful medicine too because it can protect against infections, help babies' digestion so they put on weight more easily, encourage their brain development and much, much more. You do not need very much of it at first either – just a few regular drops can do your baby a lot of good. If you can possibly give even a little, you are doing a lot more than just feeding your baby. You will be providing an important part of his medical treatment as well.

Scientists have found over a hundred different good things in breast-milk – proteins, enzymes, antibodies and other ingredients that will help protect your baby against illnesses and infections. This is particularly important for premature babies because their immune systems are not yet strong or mature enough to fight off germs very well.

If your baby is too young, too immature, or too unwell to suckle from you, and you are finding you can only manage to express a few drops of milk into a container – that's fine. A 900g (2lb) baby for example, may only be need one and a half teaspoons of milk an hour anyway, given via a tube. If you make less than this, it can be added into some formula feed. Even very small amounts of your milk can do your baby a lot of good.

Overcoming difficulties Feeding your baby on your own breast-milk in an often stressful, artificial environment like the SCBU can be hard. Whether you manage to breast-feed or not depends partly on how determined you yourself are, and on how much time you have. It also depends on how much help and support you have from the staff there.

You may not be very well yourself after your baby's birth. By the time you are feeling a bit better, it is harder for your body to start making enough milk to feed your baby. You are in an unnatural, hi-tech environment and you may be very stressed if your baby is not well.

Breast-feeding may be natural but that does not mean it is instantly easy or instinctive, even for mothers of healthy term babies. Only some 65 per cent of them try breast-feeding and only around four in ten are still breast-feeding when their babies are six weeks old. And mothers of term babies have something which really helps get breast feeding going – a healthy baby regularly suckling at the breast; most mothers of premature babies do not.

Mothers of premature babies have a great deal more than mothers of healthy term babies to cope with on just

'It was the one thing I felt I could give her that no one else could. And watching her grow and get better on my milk – that was so good.'

Claudie, Luis' mother

Giving your baby your own breast-milk doesn't mean you have to struggle to give him a hearty 20-minute breast-feed each mealtime. He may only need a couple of teaspoons at a time to get some of the very special benefits.

Breast-milk for premature babies

Research shows that the breast-milk mothers make for their premature babies is different from the milk mothers make when their babies are born at term. And the milk slowly changes too, to cater for a premature baby's changing needs as he or she becomes bigger, stronger and more mature.

Expressing by hand

1 Make sure you are warm and comfortable, and try to be relaxed. Wash your hands, and have a sterile container ready to catch your milk. Think about your baby, look at a picture of him, inhale his special scent from a piece of his clothing or blanket, or sit by him to encourage your milk to begin flowing.

2 Gently massage your breasts for a few minutes. If you are feeling tense or your shoulders are aching, ask someone to massage and knead your shoulders and upper back. Then massage your areola, the coloured surrounding part of your nipple, with your thumb above and fingers below.

3 Now try moving your entire hand firmly inwards towards your chest. Press your fingers and thumb together and move your hand away again, gently squeezing out colostrum or milk. Try to move your hand around to empty out all the different parts of your breast.

4 If the flow slows down, try changing to the other side. Go from one side to the other several times in one session.

about every front. Yet skilled and sympathetic help from the unit staff can make a huge difference. The average number of British SCBU mothers who go home with their premature babies breast-feeding is between one in ten to two in ten in Britain, yet in the units which really go all out to help you, it is nearer eight out of every ten.

Lastly, establishing breast-feeding can be a matter of time. How much can you spend on getting your milk supply going and keeping it going as you shuttle to and from the SCBU? You may have other young children to care for and the hospital may be a long way from where you live. Finding the time and peace to make breast-milk for your baby can be hard.

Expressing your breast-milk Expressing is the best way of getting your milk supply up and running – and keeping it going – until your baby is ready to breast-feed. There are many different ways to do this, and mothers usually find that there is one particular method that suits them personally the best.

There are several slightly different 'by hand' methods, small plastic hand-held pumps, some of which can be discreetly used with a shawl or big scarf draped over your shoulder, and electric breast pumps, which the hospital will have available for you to use, usually in a quiet private room. You may also be able to hire or borrow one to use at home. Some electric pumps are designed so you can pump both your breasts at once, which can save a good deal of time. Electric pumps can be very quick and efficient, but many mothers also say that they can be uncomfortable, as their suction is pretty strong. Some mothers find that they like to use the breast pump for a couple of minutes after they have hand-expressed, as this can release any milk that had been left behind more efficiently.

One of the nurses or midwives should be able to sit with you as often as you need them to, and show you how to express your milk. According to breast-feeding specialists, it works best if you begin trying to express your milk within just six hours of your baby's birth, if you possibly can. The sooner you begin, the easier it is and the longer you leave it, the harder it can be. It may not work too well the first time, or even the first few times, but it gets much easier the more often you do it.

If you have had a general anaesthetic for an emergency caesarean and are still feeling groggy, ask if a nurse or midwife experienced in helping mothers breast-feed can express your milk for you until you feel more able to start learning this gentle skill yourself. Even without a general anaesthetic, caesarian mothers need plenty of support, as the abdomen will be sore and they will need help in getting to a comfortable sitting position in bed.

If the staff do not seem really able to help you here, ask whether there is a special breast-feeding counsellor who comes in to the unit (there often is). If there isn't anyone, call up one of the breast-feeding help organizations (see *Helplines*, page 203) and ask if they have any counsellors in your area who can come and see you, either at the SCBU, or in your own home if you are back there by now.

Helping your milk supply Perhaps for the first few weeks you may only be making a little breast-milk. But as you get more and more used to expressing, you will make more. Don't panic if the amount you are making sometimes drops. This is a completely normal reaction to being worried, tired or stressed. If your milk supply is falling but you would like to keep it going, have a talk to your hospital breast-feeding counsellor (if there is one), or to any neonatal nurse or midwife at the unit who has a special interest in helping mothers breast-feed, or to a breast-feeding help organization. They will be able to advise you about the many things you can do to increase your supply.

If gentle hand massage and expressing does not help you make more milk in the usual way, some units will offer a mother some medication called Metoclopramide. It is really an anti-nausea drug, but for many women it has a useful side-effect – they find the amount of breast-milk they are making doubles. It does not work for everyone, however, and while it seems to have no adverse side-effects, not all doctors will prescribe it.

Expressing by pump

Get ready in the same way as you would to express by hand. Sometimes it helps to begin expressing a bit gently by hand first, to encourage your milk to flow. Pump until your milk stops flowing.

'Pump, pump, pump – they were constantly on at me to keep using it. I could only get out a few drops each time. It was like being a cow on a milking machine, it was so undignified. We got this little bit each day. The nurses gave Susie that down the tube and said it really was much better for her than none.'

Marine, Susie's mother

The more often you express your milk, the more you will make

Try to express every three hours during the day: some mothers have found it helps to set their watches to bleep every three hours to remind them.

You can have about five hours unbroken sleep at night without diminishing your milk supply. However, it is very important to try to express at least once during the night.

Added extras

If your baby needs anything special or extra – say more iron if he is short of it, or more calories if he has been losing weight, or more water if he is becoming dehydrated – the staff at the SCBU would, with your permission, add whatever extra is needed to your breast-milk.

Are dummies a good idea?

Some premature baby feeding experts believe that if you are planning to breast-feed your baby or are already doing so, he should not usually be given a dummy. This is because babies suck on dummies, or bottle teats, and on their mother's nipples in very different ways. So, if they practise sucking on dummies, they may not be able to breast-feed.

However, once they are upset, premature babies find it difficult to calm themselves and they use up much-needed calories crying. Sometimes, if a baby is very unsettled, and other comforting methods are not working (see page 100), having a dummy to suck on can be really helpful.

Making expressing easier Many mothers say it helps to place warm flannels on your breasts or to massage your breasts in a warm bath as it relaxes them and helps the milk to flow, though this is easier to manage at home. Sitting next to your baby and looking at him, either with your back to the room or with some screens around you so you have a little privacy, helps too. It may help to have one hand on your baby (or as nearly touching his head or body as possible) and another working a small hand-held breast pump. If you cannot sit next to your baby you may find it helps to be looking at a picture of him, or holding some clothes he has been wearing or a little blanket he has been using, and breathing in his own special scent from this. It is best to be somewhere nice and quiet: expressing milk when you are watching TV or talking to someone does not seem to work very well.

PAEDIATRIC OSTEOPATHY

Parents may also like to try to help their babies by considering some of the more well-established complementary therapies that are sometimes used to treat premature babies, such as paediatric osteopathy. This is a very gentle way of helping a baby's body achieve balance and alignment. It can alleviate the stresses imposed on premature babies by the invasive procedures they need and the equipment they are attached to. Practitioners refer to it as easing the many different disturbances encountered by premature babies in their first few weeks, and helping them back on to an even keel. A paediatric osteopath has had four years full-time training in osteopathy, plus at least two years further specialist training.

Although osteopathy as practised on adults can be a very physical treatment in which the practitioner uses firm manipulation to help realign a patient's skeleton and muscles, paediatric osteopathy, in contrast, is so gentle that a specialist practitioner may just use a single finger laid lightly against the right spot on the back of a sick 30-week premature baby's neck. Because premature babies' systems are still so fluid, practitioners only need to use the lightest touch to move a massive amount of energy. To observers it often looks as if a paediatric osteopath is doing nothing apart from gently placing a hand – or indeed a single finger – on the baby, but in fact, he or she will be making tiny adjustments. One describes it as if 'we are very subtly fitting a in small screw into a tiny hole by catching it on exactly the right thread'.

Osteopathy on the SCBU

Paediatric osteopaths work regularly on a few SCBUs, and their treatment usually relaxes and calms the babies. It can also do a lot more.

Paediatric osteopathy is often used to help premature babes with breathing difficulties. It can help clear their airways, cut back their need for extra oxygen and reduce their need for long-term ventilation help. It can even be used while a baby is on a ventilator, as long as he is stable, and the consultant in charge of the SCBU gives his or her permission. It can also be helpful in supporting babies when they are coming off certain types of drugs and medication, such as steroids and strong sedatives, which may both be needed in the first few days of life. Practitioners say that this therapy can also help reduce the profound shock which can go with IVH, and can help restore healthy blood flow.

Growing up

Paediatric osteopathy can also be very helpful for treating babies after they have come home from the SCBU. For instance, premature babies often have quite narrow heads. This may result in teething problems and mucus blocking their nose and ears, which leaves them vulnerable to coughs, colds and repeated ear infections, and perhaps hearing difficulties later on. The therapy can help their skull bones expand, encouraging the base of their skull to open out and grow as it would if they had been born at full term. It may also help, to varying degrees, with many of the health problems which premature babies can experience as they grow into toddlers and children (see *Special babies, special children*, pages 174–192).

'Nirem had gone down with a virus, his heart rate was low and he was back on the ventilator again. I could see from his neck and the whole set of his body that he didn't want to be touched – he was quite rigid. But as the osteopath started to treat him it was as if he suddenly became human again as it were, and started to respond. You could see the change in his face as he began stretching himself, smiling, and relaxing.
From that night on the nurses said he could come off the oxygen, and since then he's never looked back.'

Nishma Shah, whose twins, Nirem and Ronak, were born at 30 weeks

How to get paediatric osteopathy for your premature baby in hospital

You will need to talk to the paediatrician or neonatologist in charge of your baby's SCBU to obtain his or her permission for the paediatric osteopath to come in and treat your baby at the unit – unless, like Barnet Hospital in London, they already have a team or particular individual osteopath in on a regular basis (this is unusual in the UK).

If the consultant in charge is not familiar with paediatric osteopathy or is unsure about giving her permission, it may be worth asking the osteopaths themselves if they could possibly telephone to speak to the consultant about what the treatment involves, and how it might be of help.

Treating premature babies is a specialized area, and it is not something that every osteopath can do. To find a specialist practitioner, contact the Osteopathic Centre for Children or the General Osteopathic Council (see *Helplines*, page 203).

Cranial osteopathy

Paediatric osteopathy is not the same as cranial osteopathy. Cranial osteopaths usually just work on an individual's head and neck area and the training they have had can vary. Cranial osteopathy has however helped many babies, children and adults with difficulties ranging from sleeplessness and excessive crying (for the babies), to irritability, restlessness, headaches and learning difficulties.

To find an professionally trained osteopath who carries out cranial work, contact the the General Osteopathic Council (see *Helplines*, page 203).

Once the baby is able to suck he can take some medication – here, vitamins – through a bottle teat.

You and
your family

'I coped somehow while Jasmine was really ill, I think by just taking one day at a time. It was when she was virtually well and in the low dependency room for the last three weeks that I cracked. All the feelings I hadn't let myself feel finally hit me. I felt depressed, drained, angry, frustrated. And totally fed up. I had just suddenly had enough of all of it. I suppose I just hadn't had the space for all that before, I'd been too worried about her.'

Gillie, mother of Jasmine, whose twin brother died

Having a premature baby brings challenges and stresses to the whole family. You probably expected to be home with your baby after a few days, not having to spend weeks or months almost living at the hospital. And, while you may have prepared your older children for the arrival of a new brother or sister, they probably didn't expect to meet her wired up to a bank of monitors, or that you would be spending so much time – away from them – in the SCBU. But there are many things that can help you cope with this upheaval in your and your family's life.

WHAT ABOUT YOU?

As a mother, you may feel as though taking care of yourself is just too much to cope with, what with worrying about your baby and your other responsibilities. But, if you can possibly take some care of yourself, you will be in far better shape to help, care for and protect your baby and to look after your family. There are practical things you can do that only take a few minutes, and which could help your own energy levels and well-being greatly.

Getting your post-natal health care

New mothers of premature babies frequently miss out on ordinary medical post-natal help and care. For instance, if you have just had a baby, you would usually be visited at home for 8–10 days by a community midwife when you come out of hospital. Unfortunately, this arrangement tends to fall apart if you are not at home much because you are down in the SCBU.

One way of overcoming this is to ask for post-natal checks at the SCBU. Many units, though by no means all, can arrange for your examinations – for example to see how any stitches, from an episiotomy, a tear or a caesarean incision, are healing – to be carried out at the SCBU.

Soothing sore perineal stitches

Nearly half of all new mothers who have given birth vaginally need stitches to repair a perineal tear or an episiotomy. Perineal stitches should be feeling much better within ten days. If they aren't, this is not something that is likely to get better on its own, so ask the sister on your

SCBU unit if you can talk to one of the hospital midwives, or whether they can help you make an appointment quickly to see an obstetrician. There may be an infection, which can be healed with antibiotics, or the stitching may be too tight or have trapped a nerve, or there may be other problems which can all be sorted out by an expert.

Perineal stitches make sitting for long thoroughly uncomfortable. This is especially important for mothers of premature babies, who may find they are doing far more actual *sitting* because they are in the SCBU watching over their babies, rather than moving around freely at home.

Dealing with back pain

Around six new mothers in ten have back pain in the days or even weeks after birth, and sitting for long periods on uncomfortable hospital chairs can make the pain worse. Some of the tips mentioned here can help, but if your back is really painful or seems to be getting worse, try to make an appointment to see a practitioner such as an osteopath or chiropractor who specializes in helping new mothers. You could feel so much better after even a single session that it will be worth finding the time.

Depression and anxiety

Some feelings of depression and anxiety (often called 'baby blues') are usual even for mothers of healthy babies born at term, and as the mother of a premature baby you have difficulties to cope with that term mothers do not have. Feelings of distress and anxiety are a completely normal and reasonable reaction to the sudden, traumatic birth of a premature baby who is sick, and may be in intensive care. They should start to fade as your baby grows stronger and you are able to become more involved with her care and more confident that she will be fine after all.

However, sometimes depression can last for many months and still be there long after your baby is well and back home with you. When this happens, doctors call it post-natal depression (PND). Experts say that if PND is recognized and treated properly and promptly you can be much better within as little as three months. Unrecognized and untreated it may persist for months, sometimes years.

Making yourself more comfortable:

★ Always sit on a soft cushion.

★ Don't sit for too long at a time without a break.

★ Use the soft, old-fashioned, cotton wool-filled maternity pads for sanitary protection rather than the new ultra-thin, vinyl-coated type.

★ Wear roomy cotton briefs.

★ Find a bath you can use to have a daily warm, healing and antiseptic soak, in water with a big handful of salt added.

Relieving back pain:

★ Use a small squashy pillow underneath you or as a low back support.

★ Find something to prop your feet up about 15–20cm (5–8in).

★ Try not to sit for more than 30 minutes at a time: get up for a stretch or walk around for a moment or two, and try to do some gentle back stretching and strengthening exercises.

★ Stop muscles stiffening up and soothe discomfort with a hot water bottle, half-filled so it's pliable and can go around your lower back for about ten minutes.

★ Use some good-quality homeopathic arnica cream to rub on your shoulders and back.

Post-natal depression

★ If you have your baby prematurely you may be more likely to experience PND.

★ PND can start within the first few weeks of the baby's birth.

★ Symptoms include constant exhaustion but difficulty in sleeping, feeling increasingly detached from everything around you, worrying obsessively about the baby even if she is getting better, weepiness, irritability and anxiety.

Find someone to talk to,
for example:

★ your partner

★ a friend or relative

★ one of the nurses at the unit – anyone there you like and trust, such as your baby's 'named' nurse (the one especially in charge of your baby's care)

★ a midwife, if you are still on the postnatal ward

★ another parent on the unit

★ a parents' counsellor or psychotherapist at the unit

★ a helpline, such as Bliss, Parentline or the Samaritans (see page 203).

Recognizing post-natal depression Suspect possible PND if the way you feel is making it increasingly hard for you to cope with your daily life and/or if your baby is starting to thrive, but you are feeling steadily worse. Ask for help straight away. Tell your obstetrician or GP, or the health visitor, or one of the neonatal nurses on your baby's ward whom you like and trust, a parents' counsellor or breast-feeding counsellor, or call the Association of Post-Natal Illness helpline (see page 203).

Treatment All forms of PND are treatable, and in many cases with the right help you will be feeling much better within a few short weeks. The two main strands of treatment are counselling and medication. The latter can include hormone treatment (sometimes with oestrogen, sometimes progesterone, sometime thyroid hormone), mild antidepressants, which are not addictive, and tranquillizers, which are (though not if they are taken for less than six weeks). Tranquillizers may be prescribed if you feel so anxious that you cannot sleep and are becoming exhausted. Exhaustion makes everything, including PND, worse.

Talking

Talking about your own feelings, and having someone listen (*really* listen) to you with respect and sympathy can be healing and sanity-saving, especially if everyone has been focused on your baby's health most of the time. The things you feel are immensely important and not just because you are the central person or people in your baby's life. You have a life too.

It helps greatly if, instead of bottling up your feelings, you can find someone you can talk to.

Naming your emotions

Having a baby can produce a wild range of powerful emotions in a parent, especially a new mother: you may feel wonderful, elated, happy, and as if you rule the world, relieved, proud . . . or very vulnerable, fed up, depressed, shocked, and as if you can't cope with any of it. These feelings are all totally normal, and they do stabilize within a very few days. But having a baby prematurely can make

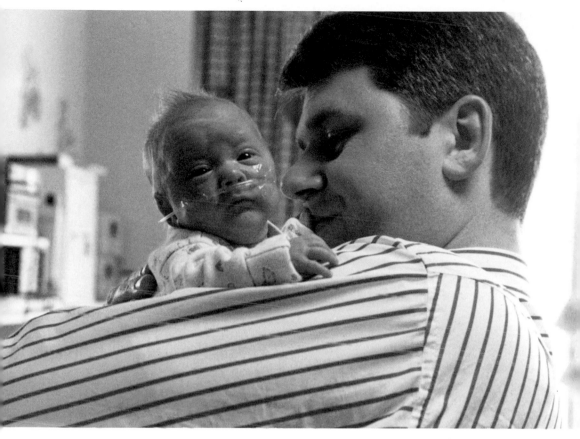

Father and baby enjoying a cuddle

you feel even more emotional, and for a good deal longer. All your powerful instincts to cuddle, feed and care for your baby in the privacy, love and support of your own home may have no outlet if your baby is so unwell you cannot hold her, or you are in a SCBU where privacy seems non-existent. On top of all that you may be very worried indeed about your child's health and even survival.

Many parents have said that recognizing and putting a name to or describing how they feel can help greatly. They also say they can remember feeling several different, powerful and sometimes conflicting emotions, ranging from blinding love, elation, obsession and hope to despair, anger, guilt and grief. They felt awe for their child, respect and pity for her as she fought for life, fiercely possessive of her, gratitude to the staff, but also powerlessness, isolation and shock, blankness and detachment, bitterness ('why

Tips for eating

★ Always eat breakfast: research shows that this helps reduce stress and depression.

★ Treat food like fuel. Live off quick and easy-to-prepare food that does the job fast and keeps you going (such as instant porridge or muesli, bananas, baked beans on toast, quick-cook pasta and sauce).

★ Buy 'healthier' takeaways that have plenty of carbohydrate in them, such as baked potatoes with fillings and a bit of salad, plus a carton of milk.

★ Buy high-calorie snack foods and frozen meals in bulk.

★ Keep some instant food (such as fruit, biscuits, instant noodles) in the SCBU unit cupboard.

★ Eat at least one square meal a day in the hospital canteen. Try to pick an off-peak time, like 12 noon before the rush starts, or 2 p.m. when it's finished. Many hospitals have meal vouchers for parents staying all day.

★ Try to drink at least a couple of litres (four pints) a day of plain water, milk or dilute fruit juices. If you are not getting enough to drink, this can sap your energy further (and it is especially important to drink lots of water if you're breast-feeding). Tea and coffee make you pee more, so you lose more vital water.

us?') and resentment of the unit staff – sometimes a mixture of these just in one short visit to their baby, and some at seemingly inappropriate times.

Eating for energy

Many new mothers of a healthy term baby find they are so busy and tired at first that they seem to be living off breakfast cereal. And they don't have to spend hours day at the SCBU, as well as possibly having to juggle care of any other older children and a home, as you may be doing. But it is important to try to eat as regularly and healthily as possible, otherwise you will not have enough energy to be very much help to your baby, let alone for any other responsibilities you may have. The suggestions on the left all come from parents who have had premature babies.

Catnapping and rest

Just 15–20 minutes of complete rest or a catnap taken between 2 p.m. and 5 p.m. has a considerable 'battery-recharging' effect. Try to find a place that's quiet and preferably off the unit for a quick but restoring mid-afternoon nap. Perhaps there is a parents' bedroom attached to the unit, or you may find that the parents' sitting room or quiet room is free at various times. Some parents kept a pillow and blanket in their car and went to lie down on the back seat for a quiet half-hour each day.

Getting help

Getting enough of the right sort of help can be quite difficult for a mother of a premature baby. One problem can be that, going home from hospital without a baby in your arms, family and friends don't treat you like a new mother who has only just given birth (and often in quite traumatic circumstances). In some cases, mothers have found that soon after they themselves came out of hospital their husbands were expecting dinner on the table, the housework done and any older children to be taken to and from school as usual.

However, many fathers want to do what they can for their partners, and may just need to be asked to do specific things – for example, your partner could be the one who makes the evening meal. This may be especially good if he does not like to spend much time at the unit itself at the moment, fearing there is nothing much he can do there for his baby (this is not true, see the previous chapter, *What can we do?*), but there is a lot he can do for you.

If you possibly can, try not to be too shy or independent to ask family or friends for a hand – nor too proud or embarrassed to accept it when it is offered. People often feel really good about being needed, and this is one time when you are entitled to all the back-up in the world. You can always return them some favours when things are easier.

If people do offer help, they may not know what sort of thing would be the most use to you. Try to give them a few suggestions, such as food shopping, a dish (such as a stew, casserole or pie) dropped in so you don't have to make a meal when you go home, picking up older children from school and giving them tea for a week, an hour of basic housework on a regular basis, or a lift to or from the SCBU each day.

Surviving in the SCBU

Just being in the SCBU for so much time can be a stressful experience for parents. It's too hot, the lights are harsh, there is constant noise from alarms, phones, buzzers, and the commotion of frequent emergencies, day and night; and there is little or no privacy.

If you feel the staff are watching you, they probably are, but this is generally because they are trying to look out for unspoken signs from parents that they might need something – perhaps practical help, encouragement, or someone to talk to.

Other parents may be watching you, too, perhaps out of sympathy because you are all in a similar difficult situation. They may just want to talk. They may be looking at you because they are very tired and feeling blank, so are staring vaguely at anything happening around them just as your eyes might stray to the TV. If your baby is ill, they may feel great sympathy but may also not know quite what to say to you.

Yet it is other parents who may come to be some of your greatest comforters and supporters at the SCBU. They

'I think I was more worried about Ashleigh. I didn't feel I could do much to help our baby at the moment. Yet Ashleigh I could help in important, practical ways. So I tried to support her by taking away the mundane tasks that she would usually have to worry about. I used to rush home from work, see her and our baby at the SCBU for 45 minutes, rush home, look after Harry, our two-year-old, tidy the house, cook the evening meal…'

Mike, father of Scarlett, born at 32 weeks

'Most of my friends had never even had a baby. They didn't know what to say to me so they didn't visit, and when they did, they'd say: "What are all those wires then?" or "Aren't you worried?" But two were great with the practicals. One gave me a lift each morning to the unit as I had no car, and my best friend did my laundry – just used to pick up the dirty stuff in the evenings, bring it back the next day clean and never even mention it.'

Maria, mother of Gavin, born at 34 weeks

'One thing we learnt was: don't go looking into the cots at other parents' babies! Respect their privacy. You may just mean to be kind in saying "hello" to a baby who looks lonely. But it's not taken well if that baby is really ill. Or even if they are not that unwell but their parents are very protective or worried about them.'

Trefor, father of triplets Tom, Ben and Megan, born at 29 weeks

'It's like being in a fish-tank. The glass around you, the humming of machines, the heat and the closed-in, hot-house feeling, and I felt like everyone knew my business.'

Maureen, mother of Nicholas, born at 34 weeks

'I have gone back to work three days a week as a nanny and I really feel like it's doing me good. The neonatal unit was my whole life for months. I have no partner to help take some of the pressure off. It's been so intense that I feel I really need another environment for a bit.'

Louise, mother of Gabrielle, born at 24 weeks

know at least part of what you feel because they feel it themselves, and are often going through very similar troubles with their own babies.

Privacy

It can be difficult to be with your baby in any kind of privacy, but it is well worth trying. Ask if there is anywhere where you and your baby could go quietly to just be together. If your partner is there, he might really like to have some peace and quiet with you both too. It can be the only time you feel you all belong together as a family.

If your baby is not well enough to come out of her incubator, ask if some screens could be placed around you both, while you sit by her.

Taking regular time out

You may find that you are spending almost all your time on the unit. You may feel fine about this; or you may find that it is exhausting you, but you feel you ought to be there. If you can possibly manage it, taking time away from the unit regularly can make all the difference between coping and not coping. However, it's important that when you take time out from the SCBU, however briefly, that you try to make it a real break. Some parents found, if they went home for a while, that unless they tried to do something specific such as watch a film on TV, they ended up sitting by the phone, worrying, instead of sitting by their baby's cot, worrying.

Try to leave the SCBU at regular intervals, even if it's just for half an hour having a drink or a snack on your own in the hospital café. If you feel up to it, go for a short walk. It is also a good idea to find places other than the SCBU where you can go regularly. If these places are in the fresh air where there is a chance of a little sun, so much the better: if you get out in daylight every day it helps your body make vitamin D (vital for healthy bones), oestrogen (to help stabilize your hormone levels) and the feel-good chemical, serotonin. Or perhaps you can find an empty room or other private space – or even go and sit in your car for a while. Larger hospitals also have chapels, libraries or gardens where you can spend some time.

Asking for changes

Because you are likely to be spending more time with your baby than anyone else, you may be noticing many things about her that the staff, who change every shift, might not. Good neonatal staff understand and respect this.

If you feel that your baby needs a change in the way that the staff are caring for her, you will probably want to say so. Parents often find it difficult to bring up anything that could be interpreted as a criticism. But remember that she is your baby, and as her parents you do have every right to ask for changes that might make things better or more comfortable for her.

You and the neonatal staff are on the same side. You want the same thing for your baby – for her to get well – and you can make a great team. Yet in the end your baby does not belong to the SCBU, she belongs to you, and it is your right to worry about your own child, to ask for things that might help her, to bring to the notice of the staff anything that you feel is the matter. Not only do you have powerful instincts as a parent, but you are not your average parent – one with a healthy term baby who has never yet had a day's serious illness. You are the watchful parent of a vulnerable premature baby.

If your early warning system is ringing but you sense that the staff might not really be listening to you when you tell them about it, you might want to look at the option of trying out a slightly different approach. Sometimes just the way a question or request is put seems to make a real difference to whether people take notice of what you say and try to help – or whether they don't.

Perhaps try saying something like: 'It would help me if you could…' rather than 'I want you to…'; 'What do you think about my baby having x, y or z?' rather than 'My baby needs x, y, or z'; 'I read this interesting idea, can I show you? What do you think about trying it?' rather than 'Experts say/this book says you should…'. Do try to comment on what was good first when you are asking for something to be changed: for example, 'When my baby had a light blanket over her yesterday she seemed much more contented. Could we try that again today?' rather

'SCBU parents are not ordinary parents. Some have been to hell and back. Some have spent days, weeks, even months sitting by an incubator, watching over their babies. Premature babies' parents understand the medical terminology, they know the complex equipment, the symptoms of many different types of disorders a premature baby can suffer from, and they know all about the treatments. Some have looked after a 2lb baby on a ventilator, others watched their children have repeated blood transfusions or even operations. Why shouldn't they worry? They have a right to. A premature baby's parent's own instinctive early warning system can save their baby's life.'

Lisa Hollis, Hospital Community Neonatal Sister at Kingston Hospital, Surrey

Being tactful

Negotiating and being diplomatic take energy. When you are tired, worried, or not yet well yourself, energy is something you may be feeling very short of, and having to be a bit tactful might seem like the last straw, but it is worth it for your baby's sake.

'I thought if I said something about every single thing I wanted to mention, they (the staff) would think I was a real pain. I didn't want the nurses not liking me much to affect the way they looked after Sam. I wanted them to like me so that they'd be specially nice with him … so sometimes I used to not say things I wanted to say, like "why has he been sitting in that dirty nappy for so long?"'

Karen, Sam's mother

'People may think you are a "fussy" parent. Well, tough. You go ahead, you have every right. I tell mothers to be like a lioness protecting her cubs.'

Anthony Kaiser, Consultant Neonatologist at St Thomas' Hospital, London

Emily holds her small brother, as their mother gives him oxygen through a funnel. The cuff on his hand is monitoring the level of oxygen in his blood.

than 'My baby doesn't like being without a covering. Where has her blanket gone?'

Try showing the nurses the things you have noticed that your baby likes. Ask if they have noticed this too. This can give you some common ground to discuss things from. Talk to other parents on the unit about what they did, how they got around certain problems. They may have found out which staff are more open to new suggestions, or found a good way through a situation similar to the one you are now trying to sort out. Ask if any of the senior nurses on the unit have regular meetings with the parents. This can be really helpful for pulling together all the information you need about how your baby is and getting certain questions answered and issues resolved, especially if you have been told different things by different people.

You need not take being told: 'No, we can't/don't do that' as permanent. Sometimes people hear something new and need to think it through, or see what you told them about for themselves, before they can understand your point. Try giving it a day or so then ask again: perhaps something like 'Do you still feel the same way about x? Perhaps you saw my baby doing y, as I did the other day? Do you have a moment to talk about it again?'

'Difficult' parents

There are a few neonatal staff who do seem to feel that a 'good' parent is someone who doesn't make any fuss: someone who doesn't ask too many questions all day, isn't around on the unit all the time, accepts what they are told and doesn't rock the boat. Don't worry if you don't conform to their no-trouble ideal of a good parent.

Feeling at home

Most parents are made to feel welcome on their baby's SCBU when they spend time there day after day, but a minority do say they notice a mixed reaction to their presence, especially if they are putting in long hours and appear to be 'always there'.

If this is the case for you and it worries you, try to have a quiet word with the sister you feel the most comfortable with. If that does not get the results you need, try talking

You need information

If you feel that the staff are becoming fed up with you because you ask too many questions, and this is bothering you, you could try saying something like: 'I know that you are finding all my questions quite irritating. But I really need information. This is my way of coping. It helps me deal with things better. For me, knowing is much better than not knowing.'

Keep a diary

Many parents do this, and say when they looked back over a couple of weeks they were usually really encouraged to see how far their baby had actually come, something that is easy to forget when you are living one day at a time.

to another more senior member of staff on the unit about how you are feeling – perhaps the psychologist, the registrar, paediatrician or neonatologist – or one of the 'supporting' staff such as the breast-feeding counsellor, social worker or chaplain.

Getting information

- Ask lots of questions – no question is too small. If you need to know something, then it matters. The chances are if you want to know about it, other parents will have too.
- If you can't catch the person you specially need to talk to, make an appointment. The sister can do this for you. In particular, trying to catch the doctor to ask important questions while he or she is on a busy ward round is not usually very effective. If you make an appointment for later, you will have some guaranteed uninterrupted time.
- Write things down (questions, points you want to mention). It can be very easy to forget bits of information when you are stressed and tired.
- Ask for written summaries of complicated information. Doctors and senior nursing staff will be happy to do this for you. (Make sure you can read their writing.)
- If you are not sure what someone meant, ask him or her to put it in ordinary words. Nurses and specialists get so used to using medical terminology amongs themselves that it is easy for them to forget that other people might find it confusing. However, parents often say they find that they do pick up the technical terms fast because they are so anxious to understand what's going on.
- Take someone with you when you are meeting the sister, neonatologist or paediatrician if you think you could do with some moral support.
- Tape information-giving conversations so you don't have to take every detail in at the time. The SCBU staff won't mind this.
- If you can't remember what a member of staff just said, it's OK to ask again – and again. No one minds. In fact, they'd be surprised if you didn't.
- Find as many books, unit information leaflets and so on as you can and read up on the subject. (Most parents find this very helpful; others don't, and some couples find they

prefer one of them to do the research while the other just focuses on coping with things as they come up.)

• Don't settle for what sounds like vague, or incomplete information; this may only make you frustrated or more worried. Neonatal staff are very busy, and you might have to push a bit to get all the information you need.

YOUR BABY'S OLDER BROTHERS AND SISTERS

Introducing even a healthy, full-term new baby to her brothers or sisters can be traumatic, touching, funny, tentative or even something of a non-event as far as the sibling is concerned. Every child's response is unique, because no two children are alike. Nor are their feelings about having a new baby brother or sister. But if the new member of the family is a premature baby who may be fragile, ill or have special needs, this may intensify the older children's natural reactions, and might, for a while, cause repeated upheavals.

Brothers and sisters' reactions may depend upon how premature the new baby is, how well or unwell she is, how well their mother is and how much time she is having to spend in hospital with the new baby every day. They may feel particularly displaced by a baby who, because she is premature, takes up so much of their parents' attention and who, as she is in hospital, may be physically removing their mother, or mother and father, from them and from their home for long periods. With older children especially, their feelings may be complicated and sharpened by worrying about the health of the new baby. Older brothers and sisters may not be any more accepting of a new premature baby than younger ones, and may miss a mother who is not able to be at home much almost as badly as a much younger child. They may also pick up more on any stress that having a premature baby is causing between you and your partner.

Helping your older children

However, at least you can often talk fairly straight-forwardly to older children, explaining the situation and finding out about how they are feeling. Let them express

'He was about the size of a newborn kitten and his chest caved inward with every breath... This baby could not live, it was impossible. I know it sounds selfish, but I knew that I couldn't stay near him. I couldn't begin to love him because if I did I wouldn't be able to cope when he died... [However,] the more I saw him the more I forgot what I had thought on that first day. He didn't really do anything and his eyes were permanently closed, but I began to feel that he was a real person, and my brother... At the beginning they fed him through a tube, but when he got a bit better we could feed him with a bottle. I came up every evening at about six o'clock to give John his bottle.'

Emily, who was 13 when her brother John was born at 24 weeks

When your children first meet the new baby

To help the meeting you might like to:

* Tape a small present to the incubator as a gift from the new baby to her brother or sister. This tends to work best with under-fives but older children may appreciate the gesture too even if they know it's from you.

* Encourage loving contact by asking if they would like to stroke the baby's head, or put a hand on her back, or cup her head without touching it, or slide a finger into her hand for her to hold, or even, if she is well enough, hold her.

* To lessen the impact of off-putting wires and tubes, explain simply what a couple of them are for, and let them trace the tube from the machine to the baby with a finger or with their eyes.

* Ask if they would like to tell a story or sing a song to the baby, very softly. Explain that she may well already know and like their voices because she got used to hearing them when she was inside the womb.

Joseph is not very old himself, and a bit apprehensive, but his little brother is safe in his arms.

their emotions and anxieties, and answer any questions they may have honestly (don't, for example, downplay the seriousness of any illnesses your baby may have), but without dwelling too much on aspects that may make them fearful. Above all, you can constantly reassure them of your love and concern for them , even though you now have another child to care for as well. Depending on how old and how capable they are, you may be able to involve them a little in their baby sibling's care, if they would like to and she is well enough.

Even if your baby's brothers and sisters are very young, there are a number of different strategies you can try to help them adjust. The advice given here is based on suggestions that parents of premature babies have said helped them with under-sevens.

Meeting the new baby

When your children make their first visit, try to welcome them on your own. It will be easier for them if you don't have the new baby in your arms or very near your side; then you can spend some loving time with them first, and all go together as a family to meet her. Some other suggestions from parents that might help this first meeting are given on the left.

Accepting the new baby

You can help your children think of the baby as part of the family by calling her by her name, and referring to her as 'our baby', 'your baby' or 'your baby sister'. To help them feel the baby is a real part of their everyday lives, encourage them to take home something of the baby's – one of her bonnets, an old hospital name tag bracelet and, especially, a picture of her – which they can keep for themselves and show to their friends. You could ask them to make a picture of the baby or colour a name sign that they could hang on the cot, and they might like to draw a picture of themselves or choose a couple of photos of themselves to leave with the baby.

There are also some books written especially for young children about premature babies (see page 203), which you could perhaps read together.

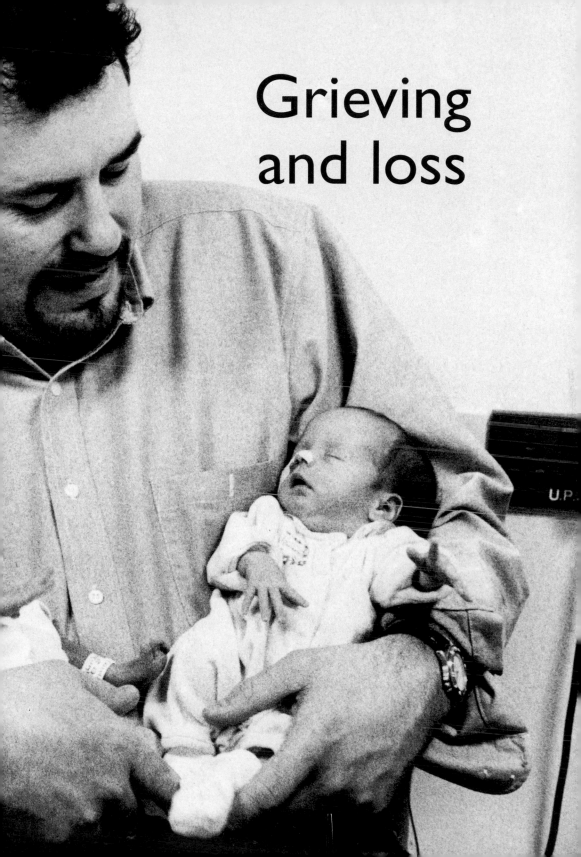

Grieving
and loss

'We had a little bedroom off the ward to ourselves and Tom was brought to us, still alive, on the ventilator. We were able to spend two or three hours with him, we dressed him ourselves, made him look nice.'

Caroline and Trefor, parents of triplets Tom, Ben and Megan.

The photograph on the previous pages shows Caroline and Trefor with Ben and Megan, after Tom's death.

Grieving for a baby with a disability

Some parents, when they find that their baby has a disability, may grieve for the child that could have been. If a baby has a serious on-going problem, the grief can be continuous, felt every time other children of the same age reach a developmental milestone which their child cannot manage: the stages at which they would usually be walking, talking, going to school, having a girlfriend, getting their first job, and so on. This grief is completely natural, too – many parents feel this way.

This chapter cannot possibly do more than touch the surface of some of the issues surrounding grieving and a premature baby's death. But we are including it in the hope that it might possibly offer something of a starting point for parents who are thinking about seeking some support for the months ahead, because they know their baby is not going to live. It is also for mothers and fathers whose babies have died.

When a premature baby does die, nothing anyone says is going to take the pain and grief away. Yet often sensitive support from family, friends, doctors, nurses or counsellors when and where you need it most, and for as long as you need it, can help you.

A premature baby who is very unwell may live for just a few hours, days, weeks or even several months. But it is not the length of the baby's life which forms the closeness: that love began in the womb. Many parents say they felt bonded with their child long before he or she was born.

THE MANY FORMS OF GRIEF

Grief is a natural response when we lose something that is important to us. That is why parents of premature babies who survive sometimes experience it. They may be grieving for what they do not have – the full-term babies they had hoped for: the babies whom they longed to have in a cot next to the bed on the maternity unit like the other mothers did, the babies who did not need to be fed with the help of tubes, the ones who came home with their parents soon after they were born. The shock and distress of having a child prematurely can be enormous, and it is completely natural to mourn like this if your baby was born too soon.

The death of a baby

Grieving for a baby who has died is especially hard. The death of a baby is so shocking that the desolation and despair can be impossible to describe. It seems completely against the natural order of things for a child to die before his parents. People who have little experience of loss sometimes think that, since there is less to remember when a baby dies, there must be less to grieve for. Yet it can be, in part, the lack of memories that makes it so hard.

The more things you have, or can recall as memories of your child, the more you will have to remember and grieve for. What one of the nurses said to you one day as they helped you dress your baby; something your baby did; the doctors' words; photographs; your baby's clothing; his hospital wrist-tag. All the small things that remind you of your child's short life and so will always be important and special.

Most of us might think that grieving takes a few weeks and that the word simply means, as it is defined in dictionaries, 'feeling deep sorrow'. But it is more comp-licated than that, and goes on for longer than most people realize. Grieving is the very personal and necessary process that people go through after they have lost someone or something they love. Ultimately it is usually a healing process, too. Every person feels different things when they grieve. These feelings can and do change from day to day, and they may last a long time.

WHY GRIEF IS IMPORTANT

Time is said to be a great healer. But it is the process of grieving, as well as time passing, that helps to heal the pain of loss. Coming to terms with loss in this way does not mean forgetting the person who died. It involves remembering, and at the same time finding a permanent and special place for that person in your life, where it does not hurt you so much.

There is no 'right' way to grieve. No one can possibly say to you: 'Do this. You'll feel much better for it.' Parents whose babies have died say that you have to find out what is right for you, then do it at your own pace. They also say that, with time, life does have meaning, purpose and joy once again, though you will never be quite the same person as you were before. They also say that it is natural still to feel and do things that you enjoy, to go out, enjoy friends' company and laugh again. But that this does not mean that you have forgotten about your baby, or that you are not still grieving inside.

Mourning that heals

William Worden, a Professor at Harvard Medical School who has worked a great deal with bereaved parents, says that there seem to be four main 'tasks' of healthy mourning.

People do not necessarily experience these tasks in any particular order, or at any specific time. They are:

1 Accepting that what has happened is true.

2 Being able to feel and express your pain and emotions.

3 Gradually coming to terms with your altered life.

4 Being able to invest energy in life again.

Most people naturally experience these tasks of mourning, in their own time, and in their own way.

'I was as tired as though I'd been working 20 weeks non-stop. I felt a terrible tense feeling inside me, almost as though I wanted to smash something up, simply because I'd lost my son.'

Adrian, whose son Rikki was born prematurely, and lived for 81 days on a ventilator

What you can do for your dying baby

Depending on how fragile your baby is and whether he is on a ventilator or not, this could include:

★ Gentle touch or massage, if your baby might like it

★ Therapeutic touch

★ Talking softly to him

★ Containment care

★ Kangaroo care

★ Just holding him close to your breast

★ Everyday care: washing, nappy changing, dressing, comforting, and feeding even if it's by tube

★ Giving your baby breast-milk, even if this is by tube

★ Staying by your baby so he can feel your presence there

★ Leaving something small and soft that smells of you, such as a small scarf, in his cot

★ 'Thinking' love and calm into him

★ Arranging for your baby to be blessed or baptized

Feelings of grief

Just some of the powerful feelings parents say they remember having when their premature babies died include anger, and unbearable pain that seemed to go on and on – many people experience this as a physical pain too. They also mentioned isolation, loneliness, disbelief ('this can't be true') and denial, numbness, frustration, deep sadness, feeling a failure, depression, anxiety, physical tiredness and lack of energy, lack of appetite, loss of interest in sex, guilt, jealousy of pregnant women, of other couples with healthy babies. These feelings can be so powerful that many parents have said they became afraid that they might actually be going mad.

WHEN YOU KNOW THAT YOUR BABY IS DYING

Mothers and fathers who were able to help take care of their dying baby have said that afterwards it helped them to feel they had done as much as they could for their child. Some parents find that caring for, and being physically close to, their dying baby feels natural, and that it is something they want to do. While for others, the fear and uncertainty create such anxiety that they pull away.

Many parents have said that they felt afraid of loving their baby when they knew he was not going to live. It is completely normal to want to distance yourself like this in the hope that it won't hurt so much when your child dies, and it can be very frightening not knowing what will actually happen. Yet it does not help to stay away. Bereaved parents have found that pulling away is, in the end, no protection from pain. In fact, the opposite is true. The less you are with your child, the more you may regret afterwards. And wishing that you had been there more with your baby can be difficult to come to terms with later.

What can mothers and fathers do?

You can do many of the things you wanted to do when you were first thinking about having a baby to care for, and certainly most of the things described in *What can we do?* (see pages 84–127). In many ways, the more you can do, the more closely bonded you will feel, which is comforting both for you and for your baby. Talk to your baby's nurses about what you might like to do for him, about what would be possible, and whether they can help and support you in this.

You might like to save some of the clothes your baby has worn, so that his scent will remind you of him at home. And it is very helpful to keep a camera and to take as many pictures of your baby as you feel you might like – perhaps photos of him with you both, with any older brothers and sisters, or with the nurses. Some parents also take beautiful photographs of their baby's small hands or feet as mementos. (Polaroids give an instant result, but they tend to fade.)

If it is possible, try to involve your baby's grandparents and close family as well, encouraging them to come and visit and get to know your baby too at this very important time. The more people know your baby, the more they can begin to understand and help you. Visiting could help grandparents themselves too, as they may also be grieving doubly – both for you (because you are their child) and for their grandchild.

WHEN YOUR BABY HAS DIED

Many parents have said it helped greatly to be able to be with their baby when he died, perhaps holding their child in their arms. Sometimes parents help to remove gently any tubes and monitor wires afterwards, then maybe wash and dress their child, or choose special clothes and other small belongings to go into the cot too. Other mothers and fathers remember they felt more comfortable when the nurse washed their baby after he had died, but wanted to come in and be with him afterwards.

Gentle goodbyes

Many have said that having a photograph taken of their baby, perhaps with the whole family, including any brothers and sisters, together – perhaps with the nurse who knew their baby best too – was very comforting to look at later on. Nearly all mothers and fathers choose to spend some time with their babies afterwards and need to

'I couldn't stop thinking about it. I went over and over the events of my baby's birth, illness and death in my mind in an endlessly repeating tape loop day after day, week after week. I couldn't stop, couldn't break out of it. I was obsessed. I thought: this is what it must feel like to go mad. I was so scared because I really thought I was going mad.'

Anya, mother of Colm, born at 32 weeks

'I have always been a fairly gregarious person; and also quite a private person emotionally. I didn't show or talk about my feelings very often. I would never have imagined I would hold or hug a dead baby. But it seemed like exactly the right thing to do at the time. It helped us say goodbye to him. We loved him so much, even though he had only been with us a couple of weeks.'

Trefor, father of Tom, Ben and Megan. Tom died in a SCBU.

Children and funerals

Although in the past children were discouraged from attending funerals, it is increasingly being recognized that this kind of ceremony can help them in coming to terms with the death of a baby brother or sister. It is important to explain to them beforehand what to expect and what will happen. This could include letting them know that people will be sad, will say prayers and sing special songs for the baby – or anything else which you feel it would help your children to know about.

have space and time in a private room. This is also a special time when you, as a mother and father, can just be parents to your child.

The postmortem

Unless the doctors are quite sure about the cause of your baby's death, they will ask your permission to carry out a postmortem examination of his body. The pathologist who performs this may be able to find out if your baby was born with any particular physical problems. This could be vital information for any future pregnancies you may have.

A postmortem is done as carefully and delicately as if your baby were having an operation. You will be able to see him again afterwards if you would like to. The procedure does not involve the hands or face, so most babies will not look very different from when their parents last saw them, except that by now their lips will probably be bluish, their skin mottled, and they will feel very cold to touch.

Some results of the postmortem may be available within a few days, others can take a few weeks. Parents are usually given an appointment in 4–6 weeks time, to meet their baby's specialist. She or he will be able to talk through any findings with you. It can be helpful to write down any questions you would like to ask as these can be hard to remember at the time. Some parents let the SCBU know when they are having this appointment so they can also then come and see the staff again for a while.

The funeral

This is a way for you to say goodbye to your baby publicly. For some parents, it's important too because it can show how much their baby touched the lives of the people he came into contact with. A funeral can be arranged directly with the hospital chaplain, with your local vicar or religious leader, or with a funeral director. Some parents choose to take their baby's body home before the funeral, which can also be arranged with the funeral director.

Feeling anxious

If your baby has lived for some time on the SCBU/NICU before he died, you may find, as many parents have, that you feel isolated and anxious for a while afterwards.

Cocooned in that environment, you are protected as much as possible by the staff and though extremely distressed at least you feel supported by people who understand, and who know both you and your baby. When you are back out in the world you can feel exposed and defenceless. It may help to know that this is completely normal, and an important part of any grieving process, but that it will pass and you will get your confidence back again.

Other people

Some friends or family members can become your lifelines. Unfortunately, others, however kind they mean to be, are not always very sensitive or understanding and may say things that hurt you (usually because they are trying to make it better) or which miss the point.

'Would he have been badly disabled? Then it was probably just as well … . ' 'But you've got two other lovely children', or 'You can always try for another baby when you're feeling better.' You may be very upset by such remarks, but try not to dwell on them. Other people may just not know what to say to you, and so avoid you for fear of upsetting you or sounding stupid.

Mothers and fathers grieve differently

The initial shock and sadness usually brings couples close to one another. But because mothers and fathers tend to grieve in different ways, the death of a child can put families and relationships under a great deal of strain as the months go by. It is very helpful if parents are able to share their feelings and support each other. When they can let each other in like this and say how they are feeling, this can help bring them close. If they cannot, there is a danger that it may tear them apart.

Fathers and mothers both feel the pain of losing their baby. But they tend to react differently and grieve for their child in very different ways. The Child Bereavement Trust have found that women usually feel better for sharing their pain and loss, for talking and crying, while men generally want to make things better, to restore and to mend. They are also usually very concerned about their partners.

Fathers often feel they need to keep away from pain, feelings and memories so they can help get things back to

'You may also find that friends and family may discourage you from doing something that you feel you would like to do. Try not to be put off. If it feels right to you, then it will probably help.'

The Child Bereavement Trust

Remembering

These are some ways in which parents whose babies have died have said it helped to keep a place for them in their and their family's lives:

* Photographs: SCBUs always have a camera and can take pictures for you or you could bring your own. Try to take as many photos as possible. Some parents find they don't want to have them at first, but feel ready to see them weeks, months, even years later.

* Keeping a treasure box of mementos, or making something in memory of your baby: a painting, a book, a little corner of garden or window box, a pillow cover.

* Thinking: perhaps there is a special quiet place you can go, a favourite spot, or a church.

* Talking to your partner about how you feel, making time to share any thoughts you have about your baby.

* Sometimes it is easier to talk things through and be supported by someone who does not know you well, such as a counsellor, a priest or, a helpline (see page 203).

* Marking anniversaries – a year after your baby's death, his birthday – in some way.

* Planting flowers or trees in your baby's memory, perhaps with a special small ceremony.

* A memorial service.

* Making an entry in a Book of Remembrance at the hospital or crematorium.

normal as quickly as possible. So, many support their wives from a practical point of view – doing the housework or shopping, taking any other children out a good deal, working to bring home the money, cuddling their partners when they cry. They do all they can to help practically, which is truly needed. But sharing the thoughts they have about their baby is needed too.

Men have often been brought up not to show their feelings. They are less likely to talk about their own emotions, and are afraid of upsetting or overburdening their partner further. They often fear that as she is so unhappy, saying anything about how they feel too may cause even more hurt. In fact, the very opposite is true.

Work is another major area of difference. Fathers are usually expected to be back at work within a very few days. Work colleagues may say they are very sorry to hear about what has happened – but then fairly quickly focus on work and the new shift/report/meeting/deadline coming up. Yet when fathers are back at home, they have to switch back into a completely different atmosphere, and often find the contrast difficult to handle day after day. For women, going back to work outside the home is usually an enormous milestone, when the only job they really wanted to have was to be at home caring for their baby.

Older brothers and sisters

It is completely natural for parents to want to protect their children from distress. But it is best to be honest with your older children if you possibly can. Parents who have been through this and professional counsellors all advise that you should explain what has happened truthfully and simply. Children tend to imagine what you don't tell them to fill in the gaps, and what they make up is usually more worrying for them. It is better to use the word 'died' rather than 'lost' or 'gone to sleep' or even just 'gone', as psychologists have found that some younger children can fear that they might get 'lost' for ever too – didn't they get lost yesterday in the supermarket? – or that if they go to sleep at night they might never wake up again either.

What your older child or children can understand will vary greatly depending on their ages and how they are told. From the age of two or three, young children can understand that their mother and father are sad because the new baby has died. But they will probably not be able to grasp the fact that death is permanent until they are older. It can help children of any age to be involved in saying goodbye to their baby brother or sister when you are all together as a family, so they feel involved and part of what has happened. Explain beforehand what to expect.

Some children find it natural to sit close to their parents and hold their dead brother or sister on their lap themselves, but offer them a choice and accept whatever they feel they would prefer to do. Many also choose to give the baby a small keepsake: ask them if there is anything they would particularly like to give. Some choose a toy they had been saving for when the baby came home.

Brothers and sisters of all ages will say their goodbyes in their own way. Perhaps by stroking the baby's head, kissing his cheek, patting his shoulder or laying a hand on the baby's tummy. They may welcome being asked if they can help choose the baby's clothes, and make the cot look nice. Some have helped a nurse take a footprint keepsake, or cut a tiny piece of hair. If one of the nurses is taking a photograph of your baby, older children often like to be there in at least one shot as part of the family.

It's fine to let your children see your tears too. They learn how to express their feelings by watching you. However, be a little wary of distressing them too much with your own painful emotions, as they may not know how to react. Children also need reassurance that you still love *them* very much, that you will still take care of them – and that you will not be this sad forever.

Your baby stays with you

Many parents find that after their baby has died, they have an ongoing and very personal relationship with him. Some say they often talk to their child in their heads, or like to go to a particular quiet spot and to remember. Mothers and fathers often say that they see their child who died as part of their family, even if he was with them for just a short time. This is normal and natural: a part of finding a way to hold on, even though you also let go.

Telling your children

It is best to be honest, and explain to children that:

★ When people die, their bodies don't work any more.

★ A dead person may look as if he is asleep but he is not, because when you are asleep your body works very well.

★ When you die, it is for ever.

★ Because our baby has died, he will not be coming home with us. This has made mum and dad very sad.

'We are still grieving for Ruqiya. I don't think grieving ever stops for parents. She's a daughter of mine. I've got three daughters. Ruqiya is the eldest and she will always be remembered as the eldest.'

Mohammed Aktar

Time to go
home

'I think the best day of my life wasn't the day Charlotte was born, as she was pretty ill and in hospital for many weeks. It was the day we finally brought her home with us.'

Sally, mother of Charlotte, who was born at 31 weeks, and developed severe pneumonia soon afterwards. She is now a healthy four-year-old.

Besides feeling joy, celebration and relief to be home with their baby at last, many parents also say they can remember feeling a bit overwhelmed at first by the sheer logistics of looking after their premature baby when they first got home. Especially if they had other children to care for too and a home to run.

For many, getting into a routine, as baby- and childcare books recommend, was well nigh impossible, and they found the easiest thing to do was to take each day as it came, abandoning housework and home-cooking until they had the strength and energy. Yet many parents remember that after a chaotic few weeks, some sort of system did develop that suited them, even though it may not have been the organized routine of the hospital or the baby manuals. All new parents feel like this, but premature babies can be hard to look after, and their parents often have much more to cope with. Remember that there are many professionals – health visitors, GPs, the community neonatal liaison sister – and helplines you can turn to for support and advice (see pages 202–3). They are there to help you: don't be afraid to ask.

Looking good

Many parents mentioned how well their babies began to look in a remarkably short time. 'She stopped looking like a pale, tired little hospital baby,' as one father put it happily. And community neonatal staff who visit mothers and their premature babies at home confirm that after about a week the babies' physical appearance tends to change dramatically. One team leader said that 'their eyes seem to sparkle, their body tone seems less floppy, they seem generally more robust, probably because they have been handled and held more. And, possibly thanks to their first bits of fresh air, their skin seems to glow.'

'We came home, I put her on the sofa then stood looking at her thinking, OK, now what do we do? It took some getting used to. But it was wonderful to be so – well, normal. I could do things like the ironing and housework, and watch her at the same time. That sounds really ordinary to other people, but because she'd been so ill and in the hospital for four months, to me just something as simple as this feels lovely.'

Louise, mother of Gabrielle, born at 24 weeks

HOW YOUR BABY MIGHT BEHAVE NOW SHE'S HOME

If your baby was born prematurely, she may at first mature at a different pace from term babies. She may also be a good deal more sensitive than a term baby for her first few weeks or months. The more prematurely she was born, the more you may notice this.

Corrected age

A baby who arrives early has two crucial dates which staff and parents use for measuring her progress. One is the day she was born, the other is her official due date, when she would have been in your womb for around 40 weeks.

The time that has elapsed from the first date is her actual age: the time from the second date is her corrected age. When you are looking at what your baby is able to do (her developmental progress) you need to think about both these dates. Especially in the first year, the gap between them can make a great deal of difference to how quickly she matures, what she can cope with, and when.

After the first year, the gap usually becomes increasingly less obvious, as most premature children tend to catch up in their second or third years. However, what a premature baby is or is not able to manage to do or cope with also depends heavily on how well she is now, how well or unwell she has been since she was born and the way she was looked after in hospital. And all babies, including term babies, have their own personal 'when I can do what' timetables, and these can vary a good deal.

Take, for example, two premature babies born at the same gestational age, having spent just 30 weeks in their mother's womb instead of the usual 40. If one of them has had a difficult time (perhaps she had repeated infections, needed an operation and was on a ventilator for several weeks) she will probably not at first develop, mature as quickly or cope with as much as the other baby who only needed tube-feeding for two weeks and had just one minor infection. The baby who was more unwell will catch up, but it may take her longer.

Immaturity and sensitivity

For some months, premature babies may not able to cope with as much stimulation from, and interaction with, their world as term babies can.

Also, a term baby's behaviour generally follows a fairly logical progression: for example, a term baby will typically

**Actual age
– Number of weeks premature**
_____
= Corrected age

You can work out your baby's corrected age from her original due date or by taking away the number of weeks or months premature she was from her actual age. So, if your baby is now five months old but was born two months prematurely, her corrected age is three months. Her level of maturity will probably – roughly – equal that of a three-month-old term baby. So she will not be able to do, or cope with, the sort of things that a five-month-old baby usually does.

'Half the time I never knew what was coming next. He'd start screaming out of the blue, fall asleep abruptly when I was trying to sing to him, cry his head off for no reason in the middle of a nice feed. Thanks to our community neonatal nurse, I eventually accepted that I wasn't doing anything wrong, that was just the way Richard was at that time. It took a good six months for him to settle down.'

Sue, mother of Richard, born at 29 weeks

Differences between premature and term babies

Every baby is an individual, but in comparison with normal term babies, premature babies newly home from hospital seem to:

★ At first, prefer less noise, less excitement, less playing with, less eye contact, and need a much calmer quieter life.

★ Find it harder to calm and comfort themselves.

★ Change their behaviour and mood, very suddenly.

★ Be more time-consuming to look after.

★ Be noisy sleepers.

All these characteristics are normal for babies born early. The earlier they were born, the more noticeable these things are.

This is because their nervous systems did not get the chance to finish developing and fine-tuning in the womb, and this process will now take a bit longer than if they were still protected inside their mothers with nothing else to do but mature.

Babies and sleep

Although babies are 'supposed' to be sleeping through the night by six months, according to the ongoing UK *Children of the 90s* survey, in reality, only 16 per cent of *term* babies are doing so let alone babies who were born early.

go from quiet sleep where she moves very little, to alert sleep where she is more active and coming close to waking up, then be awake but dozy, then fully awake and alert, then begin to fuss and cry a little and progress to full-blown crying until someone does what she needs (for example, change her wet nappy, pick her up and cuddle her, feed her). However, a premature baby tends not to follow a consistent pattern and so can be difficult for parents to care for because their baby's behaviour seems so unpredictable. She may wake suddenly screaming from a deep sleep. She may be feeding quite calmly one minute, then drop into a deep sleep with no warning drowsy period in between. Or go from feeding happily to a desperate crying fit for no obvious reason. This can make it harder to cope with or know what to do next, but it is normal behaviour for babies born prematurely, until their systems settle down.

SLEEPING

Difficulties with sleep are very common with all new babies – and with older ones for that matter – but premature babies often have particular problems, and although they may spend more time asleep than term babies, they tend to sleep for shorter periods.

Reasons for sleep problems

Premature babies have been used to the bustle, bright lights and constant noise of the SCBU. Units at night time are still very busy; and so far your baby has been trying to sleep in the atmosphere of the unit. She may be unsettled by the quiet and darkness of your home at night.

Another cause of sleep problems is that premature babies' small stomachs may only be able to take small amounts of milk at first. This does not last them long and they may wake every couple of hours needing more. By the time you have fed them, re-settled them, and got yourself back to sleep, it may be only another hour or so before they wake again.

All babies go through natural growth spurts and periods when their nervous systems mature especially fast, and the same is true for premature babies, though their timetables for doing this may be rather different. This can temporarily make a baby less settled and disturb her sleep patterns for a while.

Helping your baby to sleep

As premature babies' stomachs grow bigger and can hold more milk, and their neurological systems become more mature, they will sleep increasingly well at night. There is also quite a bit you can do to encourage this.

For instance, if your baby is unhappy with silence and darkness, leave a bedside light on near her cot to begin with, to wean her gently from wanting to go to sleep with the light full on. Later you can move the light further away, and then replace it with a dim night light. Have the radio on quietly at night, turning it down a little more each day over a period of weeks. You are trying to show your baby

A double bottle feed, at home

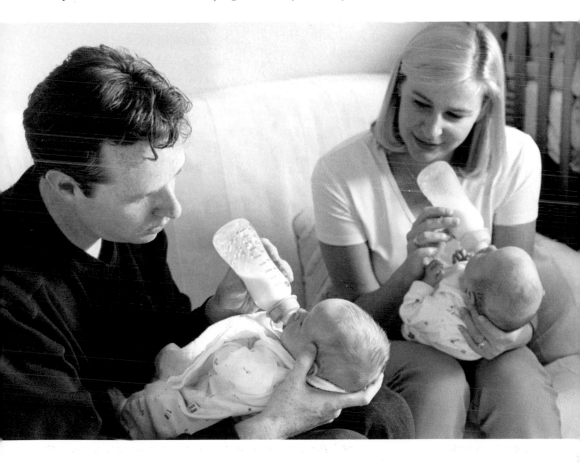

'When I took Rohan home he would scream and cry if he was in the dark, so I left a gentle night light on in the corner of the room. He didn't like it being so quiet either so for weeks we had the radio on all the time, gradually turning the volume down until there was first quiet white noise, then silence.'

Meera, mother of Rohan, born at 28 weeks

that night and day are very different (term babies need to learn this too) so during the day you might like to keep the lights on or the curtains open and a bit of background noise going and interact with your baby as much as she can cope with. At night, try to feed in a quiet, calm and cosy atmosphere and keep everything low key. If your baby needs changing, try to do this as she lies quietly in her cot rather than taking her out of it or into another room. Keep lights dim and sounds down if you can, and try to keep any interaction with your baby to a gentle minimum.

It can also help to get into some sort of routine when you are able to. It does not have to be strict, just one where certain things – a feed, a car ride to take any older children to school, a bath, a pram walk, another feed – happen more or less at the same sort of times, to give each 24 hours a bit of (flexible) structure. If you can possibly manage to do this, after a while, it will help teach your baby the difference between night and day too. Routines can have a very calming effect on the entire family. But it is far easier to establish a routine with some babies (premature or full term) than others.

If your baby often wakes with hunger, try offering a little more milk in the last night-time feed. If your baby being breast-fed but is used to occasional bottles of formula as well as your breast-milk, giving a formula feed last thing at night may help her sleep a little longer, as it takes longer to digest.

Noisy sleepers

A sleeping premature baby can make a remarkable amount of noise for someone so small – something you are unlikely to find out till you go home, unless you have roomed-in with your baby in hospital.

You do eventually get used to it though and usually sleep through it, only waking if there is a different note to the noises, for example a hungry whimper.

Minimizing your sleep disturbance

If your baby sleeps right next to your bed, flush up against the side, it is easier just to lean over, scoop her gently into bed with you to feed, then put her back into her own bed with minimal disturbance to either of you. If you do not have to get up out of bed to go to her you can do this when only half-awake and get back to sleep more easily. This is easier if you are breast-feeding. Keep basic nappy changing material by the bed too, so if necessary you can change a wet nappy as your baby lies snugly next to you (a dirty nappy will probably need a trip to the bathroom).

CRYING

Babies in general cry more than anyone thinks. At six weeks, crying for up to four hours a day is within normal limits for term babies. If you add up all the five- and fifteen-minute chunks in which crying tends to happen, even the average time is a couple of hours, which is actually quite a lot. So it is not surprising that babies who were born early, and so were that much less mature to begin with, may cry for two to four hours every day for longer than the 'usual' six weeks after their birth. Just how much longer can depend on how early your baby was born, and so how much catching up her nervous system and general development still have to do, and also on how ill she has been, how well she is now and how peaceful her environment is at home.

Crying is normal – it may even be a healthy sign. Research suggests that all babies' nervous systems go through several important stages of development in the first year of life, and it is thought that each time a baby's system goes through these developmental jumps forward, she may be more unsettled, cry more and wake up more often at night.

Calming a crying baby

There are many ways to try and calm a crying baby who was born at full term. You probably know them already. In fact, if you have other children, you are probably an expert and will have successfully used many stop-crying tactics in the past: back-patting, rocking, singing, dancing holding the baby, distraction with toys or making surprise faces.

Yet these techniques do not seem to work on a crying premature baby, even when she is well and strong enough to be home: the usual baby-soothing combination of movement, sound and sights can be too much and she will probably cry even more. Some early-born babies are overwhelmed and upset by cheery faces talking up close to theirs, being bounced up and down, or being sung to, rocked and patted all at the same time.

This may be because they are still finding it difficult to handle more than one thing happening to them at once – especially if they are already upset. Perhaps you might

Is your baby in pain?

Sleep problems and excessive crying can also be caused by medical problems. Is your baby:

* Swiping at, or even pulling at her ear or the side of her head? She may have an ear infection.

* Not wanting to lie down flat? It could be GER (see page 166) if it's after a feed, or stomach pain, or an ear infection.

* Sleeping badly, crying, and very jumpy? She may have a headache.

A headache may be something to do with her actual birth. If your baby was born vaginally, this may have compressed the soft bones of her skull a little and this compression can sometimes affect the pressure of the cerebro-spinal fluid which circulates around her spinal cord and brain. Compression may also occur if she has a degree of head flattening (see page 95).

This may produce a wide range of symptoms which can include headaches, restlessness and irritability. In this case paediatric or cranial osteopathy (see pages 124–6) may be very helpful.

Soothing tactics

You could try:

★ Wrapping or swaddling your baby and holding her comfortingly close to you as you stay still and quiet

★ 'Wearing' your baby in a sling around the house so she stays close to you all the time, or kangaroo care (see pages 102–5).

★ Resting somewhere quiet in dim light with your baby lying on your chest with her ear near the comforting, calm beat of your heart

★ containment care (see page 97).

Taking your baby's temperature

It is a good idea to learn how to do this while still on the unit. The most accurate way is using a digital thermometer: place it underneath the baby's armpit, and leave it in place for three minutes. The average normal temperature is 36.6–37.1C (97.9–98.8°F).

Checking by touch

It is also useful to be able to judge your baby's temperature by touch. Every day for a week, take her temperature, then lay your hand on the back of her neck or on her tummy (hands and feet are not accurate guides). You will soon learn to recognize what she feels like when her temperature is a bit cool, say 36C (96.8°F), or slightly raised, perhaps to 38C (100.4°F).

have already noticed that, say, sitting still and holding your baby close to you with the radio turned right down can help settle her. Yet walking to and fro as you firmly pat her back and sing her a nursery rhyme (one time-honoured way of soothing crying term babies) only makes her worse.

Crying babies with staying power can and do wear the most robust and calm parent to a frazzle. If you are worried about your baby's crying or are finding it difficult to cope with, try to get some practical and moral support. Try talking to other mothers of premature babies who know what this is like, to your health visitor, neonatal community nurse (if you have one) or GP – or, if you have very recently come home, the hospital's neonatal unit, where people will remember you and your baby. A specialist helpline like CRY-SIS or BLISS (see page 203) can also offer support and suggestions.

Try to be as flexible as you can – what works one day may not the next. And be confident that it is not going to spoil your baby if you pick her up when she cries – no matter what anyone else says about not 'giving in' to her. Most importantly, try not to feel guilty or blame yourself in any way: having a baby who cries a lot does not mean you are a bad parent. In fact, you are a really exceptional and very special parent who is having to cope with a situation that most ordinary mothers or fathers never need to handle. Most parents of premature babies have gone through more, work harder, know more, and have built up an incomparable fund of special skills, stamina, faith and patience. If you possibly can, try to make a little regular time for yourself and, so you can have short breaks, ask for and accept help. Hold on to the fact that your baby *will* settle eventually, and that in the long term it does get easier as your baby matures.

KEEPING WARM

By the time your baby comes home, she will usually be reasonably good at controlling her own body temperature. As she becomes chubbier, it is easier for her to stay warm.

Many parents worry about their babies getting too cold, as they may still seem so small and fragile, and they often have chilly hands and feet. It can be tempting to dress a small premature baby recently back from the SCBU in a thick sleepsuit, then pile the blankets or baby duvet on top of that. However, while you do not want your baby to get cold, it is equally important to make sure she does not get too hot, as this can increase the chance of cot death (see page 172).

Don't feel your house should be as warm as the SCBU, where the babies were sick. Your baby is now well enough to be be in your home. She is bigger, stronger and more mature than she was, and so better at controlling her own body heat. Generally, you should try to keep the room she is in at around 17 to 20C (63–68° F). Position her cot away from any radiators.

It is best to dress her in light layers, so that if she feels too warm to you, you can remove one layer at a time, checking her temperature after a few minutes. Be guided by how warm or cool you are feeling. If you are comfortable in a short-sleevedtop or a light dress, your baby will probably only need a cotton vest and sleepsuit with feet, a light cotton cardigan and perhaps a cotton (not nylon) bonnet.

Make up her bed, too, with several thin layers of bedding (cotton blankets and sheets) rather than a baby duvet. If you find you need a sweatshirt indoors, tuck a double layer of light cotton blanket around her.

Very small babies

If you are taking home a little premature baby who only weighs around 2,000g (4lb), she may still need to be kept a bit warmer than bigger babies. Before you go home check with the neonatologist or paediatrician as to how many layers you can safely wrap your baby up in, both in her cot and out of it.

ADJUSTING TO LIFE AT HOME

Your first few weeks or even months after bringing your baby home from the SCBU can be a bit disorienting. Most parents of premature babies remember that, at first, even simple everyday things, such as having a friend over or going to the supermarket can seem too much to cope with.

'When we first got home I had Megan in what I thought was a snug four layers of clothing, tucked up under blankets in a Moses basket. She promptly developed a temperature so I called up the SCBU in a panic. "Just take off a few layers, and take her temperature again in half an hour" said the sister calmly. I did. Sure enough, it went right back down again.'

Caroline, mother of premature Megan and Ben

Dealing with visitors

Parents' tried and tested visitor tactics include:

★ Being honest if now is not a good time.

★ Sometimes ignoring the door bell.

★ Getting a cheap answer-phone so you can choose whether or not to answer once you've heard who it is and why they are calling.

★ Asking your partner to let friends know you would like to see them (if you would) but that you are very tired, so please could they, as one mother put it: 'Take me as you find me, make your own tea, bring your own biscuits, stay half an hour at most and please call first.'

'When Scarlett was crying incessantly and Harry was playing up, getting out of the house with the pram was the thing that saved our sanity.'

Ashleigh, mother of Scarlett, born at 32 weeks

'It was all so much trouble the first few times, I nearly stayed at home.'

Vishnu, mother of Shreyas, born at 33 weeks

Visitors

Everyone handles being newly back home with a new baby (or babies) differently. However, most new parents, whether their baby was born early or at term, say they would rather not have visitors constantly popping in, as their first priority is their baby, their family, and getting their own balance back.

If visitors offer help, try to accept if you possibly can. If you find that you are too tired and muddled to think when people ask what they can do for you, keep a 'helping-out list' with, for example, shopping, cooking, laundry, picking up or taking other children to and from school, to remind you and show them what you need.

You may also find you would prefer to limit how much even the nicest visitors handle your baby. Polite discouragement tactics suggested by parents include wearing your baby in a sling close to you or securing her in a baby seat and seeing she stays there.

Out and about

It can feel like wonderful freedom and blessed normality even to do something as simple as go out with your baby in the pram after so long in the SCBU. But the sheer mental effort of getting out with your baby can also seem quite intimidating at first, especially if you are tired and have been very stressed. You may not be used to being outside much yourself, either, if you have spent weeks or months mostly at the SCBU. You may worry that your baby will catch an infection and, not surprisingly, fear crowded places such as playgroups and shops for this reason. Many mothers remember feeling overwhelmed by all the bits and pieces of equipment to take, and all the organization. Some fear the logistical difficulty of using public transport, while others worry about car safety.

You might like to wait a couple of days after coming home from hospital before you first go out. Parents often say they did this so that their babies could get used to their very different new environment before introducing them to anything else. Why not try starting small, with say, a 15–20 minute stroll to the park or round the block. Then work up to more complicated outings, for example a trip to a mother and baby clinic, or a supermarket run.

It also helps to make a list of what you might need for trips, and have essentials permanently in the changing bag and sunshades and raincovers handy for your pushchair. Leave at least half an hour after a feed before travelling by car or bus, to reduce the chance of your baby being sick, especially if she has any digestion problems.

IF YOUR BABY IS ILL

You may well need to take your baby back into hospital because she has become ill at some time during her first year at home. In fact a premature baby is up to five times as likely to need re-admitting as a baby who was born at full term. Research suggests that between one quarter and

'When Scarlett became ill I had to take her to our own GP twice and to casualty twice (all in the same four days) before she was admitted. It turned out we were right – in fact, she had pneumonia. Premature babies' parents have to trust their own good instincts about their babies. Don't be put off if the doctors make you feel like a schoolgirl being told off for making a fuss by a teacher.'

Ashleigh, Scarlett's mother

Common signs of illness

Telephone your GP or your community neonatal nurse if you notice any of the following signs, or, if you are really worried, go straight to Casualty.

1 Your baby just doesn't seem right to you – she may be behaving differently, be less active than usual, have a different note in her cry, be harder to wake up.

2 She has a temperature of over 38C (100.4°F); or a temperature raised slightly but less than this plus other symptoms.

3 She is off her food.

4 She has fewer wet nappies.

5 She is vomiting back most, or all, of her feeds.

6 She is crying more than usual, or is irritable.

7 She won't sleep, is fighting sleep, or is clearly tired but cannot seem to fall asleep.

8 She has diarrhoea.

9 She has breathing problems: pulling her chest muscles right in, breathing noisily, breathing harder or faster than usual.

10 There is a change in her skin tone: she may be paler, mottled, bluish.

11 She is limp, listless.

12 She does not like you to touch or move her. Shows discomfort when you do.

one half of all premature babies need to go back into hospital for a spell during their first year, compared with around one in ten term babies. The most usual reasons are long-term health problems including BPD, heart and digestion problems, hernia repairs and infections.

If you think your baby may be ill, trust your own instincts. If you are really concerned, take your baby to the casualty department of the nearest major hospital. Staff there should always take a potentially sick premature baby seriously, but you may need to be persistent if you sense your baby is ill but this is not yet obvious to the hospital.

Good doctors and nurses know to listen to parents, and they respect mothers' and fathers' judgment of their own baby's well-being. But if you feel something is definitely wrong yet no one is taking it seriously you may just have to nag and pester. You know how your baby is if she is unwell, you have probably seen it before, so persist.

Avoiding infection

In their first year of life premature babies are especially vulnerable to throat, lung and other breathing infections and also to ear infections. However, there are various ways in which you can reduce the risk. Make sure anyone who handles, picks up, touches or feeds your baby has newly clean hands every single time, whether they are a visitor, an older brother or sister or parents. If at all possible (though this is easier said than done), try not to take your premature baby into crowded enclosed spaces such as rush-hour buses and trains, supermarkets on a Saturday morning, packed mother and toddler groups, very busy playgroups, school classrooms and parties, at least for the first months. If you take her to the GP or clinic, try to get the first appointment of the day before the surgery fills up.

GASTRO-OESOPHAGEAL REFLUX (GER)

GER is similar to the heartburn that adults can develop. It is common in premature babies – the more premature they are, the more likely it is that they will have GER for a while.

If a premature baby has GER, the ring of muscle that separates the stomach from the oesophagus (gullet) is too weak to remain closed, as it is supposed to. This means that partially digested milk and burning stomach acids can find their way up from the stomach where they belong, into your baby's throat. This is called regurgitation. When a baby regurgitates because she has GER, she may also gag, stop breathing for a moment, then start coughing and choking. This tends to happen (if it is going to) during or after a feed or when your baby is lying down asleep, especially if she is on her back.

GER can be miserably uncomfortable and, in some severe cases, if it has not been spotted and treated, the baby's oesophagus can develop painful ulcerated patches. GER can also make it difficult for a baby to feed happily or to keep her milk in her stomach afterwards. This then makes it harder for her to gain weight or grow well.

If it is not tackled, the regular discomfort of GER each time she feeds may also make it generally difficult for a baby to enjoy eating. It may even create a dislike or in extreme cases a fear of eating and swallowing food that may carry on well into toddlerhood and early childhood.

The good news about GER

GER tends to disappear as your baby spends more time upright – first sitting up alone, then toddling and walking. This is partly because her overall muscle-tone is improving, including that of the ring of muscle separating stomach from oesophagus; and partly because, as she remains more upright, gravity helps to keep the food down instead of allowing it to come back up.

What parents can do to help

In general, if your baby has GER, it helps to keep her as upright as possible most of the time. Try walking around holding her against your shoulder, or sit with her lying up against your shoulder on her tummy. At night, you could try semi-reclining in bed with your baby stretched out comfortably on her front with her head on your shoulder and feet pointing down towards your waist.

If you possibly can, try not to focus too much on your baby's weight gain at the moment. This can be a really major worry for parents whose babies have GER. Yet if

Managing GER

★ Feed your baby with her sitting upright or at least semi-upright and make sure she stays upright for about half an hour after each feed.

★ Feed slowly, taking several breaks and rests; or feed her less milk at a time, but more often.

★ Add a thickener such as Carobel to her feeds. Ask your neonatal community sister, GP, baby clinic or health visitor about this.

★ Change your baby before, rather than during or after, her feed and make sure her nappy is not too tight around her stomach.

★ Raise up the head end of your baby's cot or basket so it's at about a 30 degree angle. A baby buggy whose sleeping position you can adjust to the same angle may be very useful here too.

★ Check your baby does not have problems digesting milk protein (milk intolerance). Ask your GP, paediatrician or neonatal community sister about this.

★ If your baby is bottle-fed, check to see whether the formula milk powder you are using is based on casein. Some health experts recommend this should not be used for premature babies even when they get older, as it can be hard to digest.

Signs of possible breathing trouble

If your baby is:

★ Breathing faster than usual (approximately 60 or more breaths a minute)

★ Having to work hard to breathe, pulling her chest in very noticeably (doctors call these retractions)

★ Wheezing

Any of these may signal the early beginnings of a breathing infection. See or speak to your GP that day. If he is not helpful, or your baby becomes worse, call him again, or go to the Casualty department of your local hospital.

The National Asthma Campaign's tips may help snuffly premature babies. Try:

★ Damp-dusting all surfaces

★ Washing any removable furniture covers

★ Washing any furry household pets, especially cats (difficult to do, but many asthma specialists believe that cats, and to a lesser extent dogs, are asthma sensitizers)

★ Keeping a runny nose clear by using a soft tissue

'When the SBCU first suggested the idea of taking Mark home while he was still oxygen dependent, I thought – I don't know, I'm not a nurse. I can't do this. But we did. And it was the best decision we ever made.'

Catherine, mother of Mark, born at 32 weeks, who had chronic lung disease

your baby is otherwise well, and being monitored by both you (who know her best) and good health professionals, you are doing all you need to at the moment. See if you can handle the GER by gently managing the way your baby feeds or sleeps, because that just may be all you need. But if you feel that some medical help is called for, see your GP or baby clinic. They will probably prescribe a medicine to reduce the levels of acid in your baby's stomach and/or one to speed up the rate at which it empties itself of food (so there is less sitting there waiting to come back up again).

BREATHING PROBLEMS

In their first year at home, premature babies tend to have more respiratory (breathing) infections than term babies. If your baby has had BPD and needed to be on a ventilator or had long-term breathing support she will be more vulnerable to this type of infection. Colds, blocked noses, coughs and sore throats can be thoroughly uncomfortable and may interfere with sleeping or feeding, but they are usually not serious. Occasionally, however, what appears to be a minor infection can develop into a more severe illness, such as bronchiolitis or pneumonia, so it is a good idea to keep a careful eye on your baby if she does get a cold. Breathing infections are among the most common reasons for readmitting former SCBU babies to hospital during this first year.

The snuffles

At the milder end of the scale, premature babies are often very snuffly when they first come home. This could just be a reaction to ordinary house dust and should pass in time as your baby gets used to dust mites and stray pet hairs..

If your baby seems to be otherwise healthy and is feeding well you can ignore persistent snuffling for the moment and carry on as usual. But if she has had support from oxygen therapy at home (see below) and develops this type of condition, keep a close watch. If she develops a respiratory infection, even a cold, she may need oxygen therapy again for a while to help her recover.

COMING HOME WITH OXYGEN

Babies who need extra oxygen but are otherwise well, stable and have reached a reasonable weight may be allowed home if their parents can learn and feel confident about the care and equipment they will need.

A premature baby may need this extra help for just a few months but in some cases the time-scale is a few years. This may sound a bit daunting, yet most parents who have done this say they did not find many problems with using the equipment once they become used to it. The SCBU staff will show you how to operate the oxygen machinery until you are confident with it, and arrange for it to be installed at your home.

Once you are all home, a community neonatal nurse or other specialist health professional will visit you regularly to support you and help with any difficulties you may experience. They will also assess your baby regularly, to see how she is doing and whether the amount of oxygen she is being given can be gradually reduced.

You would probably be using either oxygen cylinders, or a device called an oxygen compressor or concentrator which separates the oxygen out of air and feeds it to your baby. As the concentrator runs on electricity, you would also have a portable back-up oxygen tank to use when you are out and about, or in case there is ever a power cut.

Parents and their premature baby often share a room attached to the SCBU for a night or two, before they all go home together, so that the parents can become used to being 'in sole charge' while still having the reassurance of knowing the staff are there if they need them. If your baby is going home still needing oxygen, you might like to room in for a couple of nights or so to give yourself time to become comfortable with using the cylinders or compressor too.

The most common reason for a premature baby to graduate from the SCBU to her home still needing oxygen support is that she was born before 32 weeks and has BPD – chronic lung damage (see page 61). The good news is that as your baby grows so does new lung tissue, and the damaged lung will often heal.

The benefits of home oxygen therapy

If a premature baby needs oxygen therapy, it can sometimes be a long time – up to as much as four years from the time she began – before she is weaned off extra oxygen completely. Giving her oxygen yourself means that, rather than spending that time in hospital, your baby is at home where you can be a family together. Premature babies thrive and grow better, are happier, feed better and are less likely to pick up infections at home than they would in hospital. And you won't have to be constantly torn between being at the hospital and home.

Oxygen therapy: cautions

★ Oxygen is highly flammable. Keep your baby well away from any open flames, such as an open fire or a gas appliance with a pilot light.

★ No smoking in the room where the oxygen equipment is kept.

★ Keep your baby away from smoky atmospheres.

★ Make sure your home is fitted with smoke detectors – and that they work.

★ Keep the door of the room open so it does not become stuffy.

Weight gain – how much is enough?

'Ideal' weight gain for a new baby is about 28g (1oz) a day, but a premature baby may not be putting on this much, especially if she has a condition affecting weight gain such as BPD (see page 61) or GER (see page 166).

Talk to your paediatrician or neonatologist about the sort of weight gain they feel is enough for your own baby. Check how much weight she is putting on using a centile chart. You will find one of these in her medical records, and also in the home baby book record of health. If she is below the bottom centile (that is, the band with the lightest weights) but running parallel to it rather than dropping away, that's usually enough.

Common tube problems

★ Irritation, soreness or a little bleeding around the nostril the tube goes into. A little petroleum jelly can help protect against this. The tube can also easily be changed over to the other side while the sore nostril heals.

★ Occasionally the tube may cause irritation or soreness in the gullet. If you do notice a little blood (perhaps when your baby brings up some milk) let her doctor know.

★ When the tube is put in or removed, it may make a baby gag, or vomit briefly.

If your baby regularly becomes short of oxygen after feeding, or after other activities , such as being bathed, she may also go home with temporary oxygen support.

When your baby is having oxygen therapy you need to keep a very careful eye on her if she has a respiratory infection. Ask your GP about flu vaccine for her too and make sure that her whooping cough vaccination course is completed on time.

FEEDING YOUR BABY BY TUBE

Usually by the time a premature baby is well and strong enough to go home, she will be taking as much milk as she needs for herself, whether it is from your breast, from a bottle or from a special feeding cup (see page 116).

However, some babies are not able to do this just yet. This may be because they have heart or breathing disorders, a problem with their oesophagus, because they still cannot quite manage to co-ordinate their sucking, breathing and swallowing, or because they get very tired before they finish their feeds. If a baby is not yet taking enough nourishment by suckling or drinking, she will also have her calorie levels regularly topped up with tube-feeding. Once babies have reached a certain size and are otherwise well enough, it may be possible for them to go home in spite of their needing tube-feeding. Different SCBUs have different policies as to how big is big enough to go home.

Using a naso-gastric (NG) tube at home

If your baby is being fed in this way (see page 114), try to let her suckle on your breast or her bottle (if she is able to) as much as she can for the first part of the feed. Then attach a small syringe filled with the rest of the bottled milk or with some of your own expressed milk that has been waiting warmed and ready next to you and feed it to your baby slowly by gravity flow.

Other forms of tube-feeding

Some babies cannot use an NG tube because it does block part of one of their nostrils and can make it more difficult to breathe. If so, an oro-gastric (OG) tube, which goes into the mouth, may be used instead. It is usually put in carefully before feeding and removed afterwards each time. The taking out and replacing of the OG tube can upset babies, however, and may make them gag or vomit.

HERNIAS

A hernia is a small loop of intestine that has managed to push its way through a weakness in the muscle of the baby's abdominal wall. It usually looks like a firm lump on the skin's smooth surface. Hernias are surprisingly common in premature babies, and will often disappear on their own. If a hernia appears in the baby's groin, it is known as an **inguinal** hernia, if it appears behind the baby's belly-button, it is an **umbilical** hernia.

Umbilical hernias tend to sort themselves out without any treatment, and have often vanished by the baby's first or second birthday. If it does not, the baby may have an operation to repair the small gap in the abdominal muscle wall. Inguinal hernias, which are far more common in boys, will often be repaired while babies are still on the SCBU, as soon as the doctors are confident that they are mature enough to tolerate an anaesthetic.

There is also a very small chance that any hernia may strangulate. This means it twists and cuts off its own blood supply. Signs of a strangulated hernia include the lump darkening or becoming bigger or tender to touch, vomiting and severe colicky pains.

If you see any of these signs, ring your GP right away, because if the hernia has indeed strangulated this a medical emergency. It can, however, be repaired very successfully with a prompt operation.

HELPING PREVENT COT DEATH

When a baby dies suddenly and no one can find the cause, this is called cot death, or Sudden Infant Death Syndrome (SIDS). Fortunately, cot death is relatively rare now (it affected 469 UK babies in 1997) and often preventable. For instance there has been a campaign running since 1991 called 'Reduce the Risk' which promotes putting babies to

Hernias in premature babies

★ Can affect up to one in four premature babies.

★ Are far more common in boys.

★ The less a baby weighs at birth or the more premature he is, the likelier he is to have one.

★ A hernia lump may appear to come and go. It can be especially noticeable if the baby is crying hard.

Helping to protect your baby from cot death

★ Outlaw smoking from your house. If you don't smoke and you don't let anyone else smoke anywhere near your baby, you reduce her risk of cot death sevenfold.

★ Put your baby in the feet-to foot sleep position – that is, with her feet right down at the end of the cot so she can't wriggle under her bedding and risk covering her head.

★ If you are at all worried that your baby is not well, go ahead and ask for help immediately. Health professionals give number one priority to premature babies who have recently come home. If you are worried that after repeated phone calls from you they may think you are fussy parent, so be it. Being a fussy parent could save your baby's life.

Trying to stop smoking

If you are a smoker, try to cut down, or better still give up altogether if you possibly can. Babies, especially premature babies, and cigarettes do not mix.

Unfortunately, giving up cigarettes is easy enough for health professionals and books to suggest but in the real world it can be very tough to do, because tobacco is so addictive. Also, you may never have felt more like smoking in your life. Having a premature baby can be very stressful, both when she is unwell and being cared for in the SCBU and when she is back at home with you. But not smoking is such a vital part of keeping your baby healthy that it is worth trying hard to stop. (See *Helplines*, page 203).

sleep on their backs rather than their fronts and this alone has cut the SIDS numbers by half.

Parents of premature babies often worry about cot death. Your baby was extremely well protected in the SCBU where staff monitored her health continuously, and were on hand immediately whenever there is a problem. Now your baby is well and strong enough to go home with you, she will have her own much improved health and strength – and you – to help keep her safe and this will nearly always be all she needs. However, premature babies do run a higher risk of cot death, and there are several important steps you can still take to protect them from this (now very small) possibility.

How warm should my baby be?

It is important to make sure that newborns and young babies do not get too hot, as that can increase the risk of cot death. See pages 162–3 for advice on how warm you should keep your baby.

Sleep position

Putting newborns to sleep on their backs has halved the number of cot death babies in the UK, and this may well be the safest position for your baby. However, the Foundation for the Study of Infant Deaths (FSID) says that for some premature babies – such as those who have particular types of breathing problem – this may not always be suitable. They advise talking to your neonatologist or paediatrician about the best and most comfortable sleep position for your baby.

Alarms

If your baby's specialist advises you to let her sleep face down (prone), head to one side, and you are concerned about this, talk to him or her about whether hiring or buying a baby alarm monitor for use at home would be helpful in your baby's particular case. The FSID also have useful information they can send you about baby alarms (see *Helplines*, page 203). There are two sorts. One detects your baby's breathing pauses, the other goes off if her heartbeat becomes too slow. Either may be part of a sensor pad that a baby lies upon, or attached around her middle with a special belt. Both are very different from the walkie-talkie style baby monitor devices where you leave one handset in your baby's room and take the other with you – these are just listening-in devices so you can hear your baby cry if you are in another part of the house.

However, these alarms may be more trouble than they are worth. Parents have reported being reduced to nervous wrecks by the number of frequent false alarms. One major survey in *Which?* magazine found that seven in every ten mothers gave up using the monitors because of this. Other parents say they became so dependent on the reassurance the monitor gave them they were afraid to go anywhere without it and so hardly ever went out at all.

The FSID also points out that the alarms do not always detect trouble because sometimes they may not go off at all, or go off too late. For instance, though this is rare, if your baby's windpipe becomes blocked she may carry on making breathing movements and the alarm will not sound – but she can still suffocate. Another reported problem is that because the alarms have a pre-set time before they ring, they may not go off in time: though with a 20-second alarm, you do in practice have minutes in which to act, rather than seconds.

Breast-feeding

Premature babies, are still extra vulnerable to catching bugs of all sorts for many months, even when they are well enough to go home, and infections are a risk factor in cot death. Breast-feeding your baby gives real protection against infections, and so will help keep her safe.

Firm cot mattress

No one has yet found a type of mattress that actually protects against cot death. But it is best to use one that is firm, in good condition (get rid of it if it seems to be deteriorating), clean, dry and well aired. The FSID also recommends that babies should have no pillows or padded cot bumpers until they are at least a year old, because they might increase the risk of your baby overheating in bed.

'The monitor ruled our lives. It used to sound several times a day and each time my heart was in my mouth as I ran into her room. I found I could never relax, I kept expecting it to go off again any minute. But I would rather run to her a thousand times over for nothing than miss the one time when it was for real...'

Kim, father of Kirsty, born at 33 weeks

Emergency measures at home

If the alarm does go off, and you go quickly to your baby to find that she does need help, would you know what to do? Ask your baby's nurses to show you how to resuscitate your baby just in case you should ever need to, before you go home together; or, if you are already at home, ask your health visitor or GP to show you.

Special babies,
special children

'We are very optimistic indeed about premature babies who are born from as little as 31 weeks. Most either have no on-going problems at all, or if they do they tend to be very short term.'

Andrew Whitelaw, Professor of Neonatal Medicine at the University of Bristol and an international expert on the care and development of children born prematurely

'First it was a roller-coaster of: is he going to live? As he got better, it was: when can we take him home? Then, when we were all home, it was: how is he going to get on as he grows up? Is our son going to be normal? Now [at nine] he's already 4' 11", has his first two belts in karate, a wicked sense of humour, and is in the top set at school for everything except French ... '

Mandy, whose son Christopher was born at 28 weeks, developed pneumonia then had a moderate IVH episode

Most premature babies now grow up fine, with no lasting physical or mental problems whatsoever. Research shows survival rates for babies of 31 weeks (gestational age) and over to be upwards of 98 per cent. In fact, overall, most babies born as early as 26 weeks will go on to do well.

Part of the reason for this is the now standard hospital practice of giving steroids to mothers who are in, or look as if they may begin, premature labour. This helps mature the lungs of their unborn babies while they are still in the womb. More mature lungs mean easier breathing when a baby is born, and easier breathing means a better supply of oxygen to the brain. This is especially important because if the brain's supply of oxygen is interrupted or reduced, it can be damaged quite quickly. This damage may be very slight, but it can be substantial.

Another treatment that has improved premature babies' ability to breathe – and therefore their overall health and ability to survive without developing difficulties – is the practice of giving them surfactant replacement (see page 60).

Over the last two decades there have also been enormous improvements in high-tech life-support equipment for premature babies, such as sophisticated ventilator machines. In addition, there have been valuable advances in the methods of monitoring babies' blood pressure and blood oxygen levels, and huge improvements in the treatments for the type of problems premature babies are especially vulnerable to, from IVH and heart defects to infections.

POSSIBLE PROBLEMS

Most premature babies have no disabilities or ongoing difficulties at all. But it is also true that the earlier they were born, the more likely it is that they may have a problem. For most babies, the problem will either be a very mild one that is barely noticeable, such as squint, or a moderate difficulty, perhaps problems with co-ordinating movement, which will respond well to physiotherapy support and other treatments. But in a small number of cases, the disability may be more severe.

What is a disability?

Disability and handicap are words that are used very loosely. But in general they describe any physical or mental problem that prevents people from doing the things they would like to do for themselves, or which restricts the way they live.

Doctors divide disability into three grades: mild, moderate or severe. A severe disability means that the person needs physical help from someone else to manage his ordinary, everyday activities such as eating, washing, getting dressed or going out and about. Blindness, when someone can see nothing or only light or dark, profound deafness, severe cerebral palsy, and an IQ (see page 188) of below 70 points are all seen as potentially severe disabilities or handicaps.

Will my baby have a significant problem?

Professor Whitelaw estimates that the likelihood of a baby having a significant disability is about 10 per cent if he was born at 28 weeks, and 20–30 per cent if he was born very early, at around 24 or 25 weeks.

For four years a major British study called EPICure (1999) followed some 300 babies who were born extremely prematurely – that is, before 26 weeks. Published results show that about half (51 per cent) had no problems at all. A further quarter (26 per cent) just had mild to moderate problems, such as a hearing difficulty which could be corrected with a discreet hearing aid, short-sightedness which could be managed with the right pair of glasses, or a mild weakness in their legs which did not even interfere with their walking.

However, the remaining quarter (23 per cent) of the children did have severe disabilities. These included significant cerebral palsy, major developmental delay, seizures, hydrocephalus which needed a permanent shunt (see page 72) and blindness.

Factors influencing the likelihood of disability

Apart from being born extremely early (before 26 weeks), there are also other factors that make it more likely that a baby might have a disability. If your child has experienced

Risk factors for disability

These include:

* Being born before 26 weeks

* Becoming very short of oxygen while being born (birth asphyxia)

* Bleeding in the brain (IVH)

* Severe jaundice

* Very low levels of sugar in the blood in the first few weeks of life (hypoglycaemia)

* Chronic, long-term illnesses (such as broncho-pulmonary dysplasia)

* Severe infections, such as those caused by herpes and Group B streptococcus

* A long and difficult stay in a NICU

* Having needed long-term ventilator support

The difference parents can make

'If a baby has a problem, parents can do a huge amount to help. I can still remember one particular little girl who was born prematurely and then had an intra-ventricular haemorrhage which all but devastated one side of her brain. But she was lucky enough to have terrific parents. Thanks to her mother, a Greek Cypriot, and her father, who was Polish, this little girl did so well that she was speaking three very different languages – English, Greek and Polish – by the time she was three.

I have worked with several families like that, and have seen this happen again and again. This is why I know that parents' love, encouragement and stimulation can make such an enormous difference: because, at that age, a baby's brain is quite plastic. It can be very adaptable because it is constantly making so many new neurological connections while the child is still very young. So if one side is damaged, the other side can often take over.'

Andrew Whitelaw, Professor of Neonatal Medicine at the University of Bristol

At almost three John is still very small, but he is growing up fast.

any of these, it makes good sense for him to have his sight and hearing checked by hospital specialists before he leaves the SCBU, and to have regular developmental check-ups in the hospital follow-up clinic. This will help ensure that any problems will be noticed as early as possible. The sooner problems are detected, the more successful treatment and help will be.

A baby's home environment

A premature baby's home environment also has a great influence on the outcome of any problems. A good home environment has nothing whatever to do with wealth or privilege. It doesn't mean having a big, smart house or expensive toys. It means having loving, positive parents (or a parent) there who are consistently doing the best they can to encourage, care for and stimulate their baby in appropriate ways as he grows up. When a baby does have a good home environment, this can go a long way towards reducing the effects of many developmental problems.

Parents make a big difference

The impact of a baby's parents and his environment on his development cannot be emphasized enough, according to TrezMarie Zotkiewicz, Neonatal Discharge Co-ordinator at the Ochsner Foundation Hospital in New Orleans. 'Infants with known developmental risks such as IVH may develop normally with early intervention and appropriate stimulation at home. Yet babies discharged as "well" may return to follow-up clinics with significant delays, in part because of lack of learning opportunities at home.' This view is shared by most neonatal experts.

FOLLOWING UP YOUR BABY: CHECKING AND SUPPORTING

When you go home with your premature baby, you need not feel alone. There are many health professionals and parents' help groups there to support you, and a big cast of specialists who can assess and help with your baby or child's development (see pages 202–3).

At your baby's follow-up clinic, you will meet the team who will monitor him after he leaves the SCBU to go home

Worries

If you are worried about something, **you do not need to wait until the next check-up appointment** to discuss it. Ring the follow-up clinic, your GP or health visitor, or your community neonatal liaison nurse if you have one.

with you, and support you if you have concerns about his health or development. Please see *Caring for your child* on page 202 for who is likely to be in the team. Their job is to check your baby's developmental progress (his speech, hearing, movement and so on) and his physical and mental health at regular intervals, as he grows up into toddlerhood and beyond. If any difficulties arise, the team will be there to help diagnose and treat them.

Parents say that it is very helpful and reassuring to develop a good relationship with the follow-up clinic, even with just one of the team there – perhaps with the paediatrician, or a particular member of staff with whom you feel especially comfortable. This can make asking questions and mentioning any concerns you have much easier. It is also really important to go to every single follow-up appointment, whether it is a standard developmental check with your health visitor or a date with the hospital audiologist to check your child's hearing.

Follow-up checks

Most neonatal follow-up units will see a child who was born at 30 weeks or less at regular intervals until he is about two years old. If he has a particular problem, a community paediatrician will keep an eye on his progress for longer. In addition, he may be referred to a specialist, such as a respiratory paediatrician if he has long-term breathing difficulties.

The timetable of your baby's check-ups will vary depending on your hospital or local health authority's policies, on how well or unwell your child has been, on whether he has any particular problems and, if he does, on how severe these are. But the following is an example of the basic type of check-up schedule your child may have. Some of the stages depend on your baby's corrected age – his age counted from the day he would have been born if he had not arrived prematurely (see page 157).

The first visit One to two weeks after going home with your baby, you may have a first visit from a community neonatal nurse (if your area has one). These visits can continue once or twice a week if you need them, for between six weeks and a year, depending on your child's needs and also on the area's policy and resources.

Six weeks (corrected age) Your baby will have his first assessment from your GP and/or health visitor.
They will check your child's:
• movement and reflexes
• sight
• social development (Is he interested when you talk to him? Does he smile yet? Follow you about with his eyes?)
• hearing
• hips, as these may occasionally have been dislocated at birth
• weight, length and head size (its circumference)
• testes (if he is a boy) to see if these have descended (dropped) yet

Immunizations Your doctor or health visitor may also want to discuss immunizations with you. Most health professionals will prefer to give a premature baby the standard immunizations at the usual times, and will not take your baby's corrected age into account. The exception is the polio immunization which, as it is a live vaccine, will not be given when he is still in hospital.

Four months Your baby will have his first developmental check-up at the hospital follow-up clinic, to assess neurological and general development. The clinic will have specialists in many different aspects of the physical and mental development of young children. The four-month check is also a good chance to talk about anything at all that you may be worried about, however small it might be.

Seven months The hospital follow-up clinic will check neurological and general development and give your baby a hearing test.

Eight months The health visitor or GP (usually the health visitor) will check the same things that they did at six weeks, as well as checking what sort of sounds your baby likes to make at the moment, as these are a prelude to learning to talk. They may also do another hearing test.

Asking for specific information

Parents whose premature babies are now growing up say that it is helpful to try to get very specific answers to a few questions at every clinic visit – for example:

★ When will I know about x?

★ What does it mean if we see our child doing y?

★ How long will he need this therapy for?

★ When might we expect to see the therapy helping?

Then at least you will come away with some concrete information every time.

It may help to write questions down before you see the follow-up staff, and also to take notes of their answers.

Twelve months The hospital follow up clinic is likely to carry out a detailed assessment of your baby's development. At this stage he may have other appointments or be referred to a specialist, depending on whether or not any particular problems – perhaps with hearing, vision, movement, or feeding – have come up.

Twelve to eighteen months The health visitor will do a developmental check on all the things she looked at before, as well as checking your child's speech.

Three and a half years The health visitor will give your child a pre-school development assessment.

YOUR CHILD'S DEVELOPMENT

Neonatal experts and parents whose premature babies are growing up into toddlerhood and beyond all say that it is best not to expect a smooth, textbook development. All babies have their own individual timetables for doing things, and this is especially so for premature babies. Long-term illness, a difficult stay in hospital, an ongoing health problem or a disability are all things that may slow down your baby's progress.

It is hard not to make comparisons with other children who were born at term, or when reading baby-and-childcare books, but try to bear in mind two important things: your child's corrected age and the fact that most premature babies do 'catch up', but in their own time. Parents say it is very encouraging to keep a diary of all your child's steps forward and achievements and that sometimes when thay look back at it, they are amazed and comforted by how far their children have come.

Growth

A child's growth is affected by many different things. These include how well he is, how much he weighed when he was born, how early he was born, genetics (the things he inherits from you, his parents), whether he needed special care at an NICU, of what sort and how long he stayed. Other important factors include the sort of health problems your child has had so far, how he was cared for in hospital, and how he is looked after at home.

Babies weighing more than 1,000g (2lb 3oz) at birth will usually have more or less caught up by the time they are four or five years old. But, babies born weighing 1,000g or less will take longer to reach their growth potential (that is, the best growth they can achieve). However, with the high-calorie milk formulas now available, most babies who were born prematurely are now reaching their growth potential faster than they did ten years ago.

Action Keep an eye on your child's weight and height using the growth charts in the health record book that all new babies have. You will be given one of these books by your health visitor, by your GP, by a mother and baby clinic if you are going to one, or your child's follow-up clinic at the hospital. If you have any concerns at all, for example worries about feeding difficulties, either your community liaison neonatal sister (if you have one visiting you) or the staff at the follow-up clinic can help advise and support you.

Parents are often worried about whether their child is growing properly. 'Try to look at the rate at which he is growing, rather than how big he is,' suggests Neil Marlow, Professor of Neonatal Medicine at Nottingham University. 'If a child is growing at a normal rate, then he is probably fine, even if he is smaller than other children of his age who were born at term.'

If he is not growing at a normal rate, contact your community paediatrician. He or she will probably want to examine your child carefully and perhaps carry out some tests to see if there is any reason for this. It is not likely that a specialist would give your child treatment with growth hormone these days, despite the amount of press coverage it has had over the years. This is because, according to Professor Marlow, the gain in height that it gives is only short term.

Sight

Around a quarter of babies born weighing less than 1,000g (2lb 3oz) will have some sort of difficulty with their sight, but this drops sharply to just 2 per cent for babies weighing more than 1,000g.

Premature babies who were born at 34 weeks or later and were the right weight for the amount of time they have spent in the womb (doctors may use the term *appropriate for gestational age*, or *AGA* to describe this) will usually grow at around the same rate as a term baby.

One of the vision problems that often affects very premature babies is retinopathy of prematurity or ROP (see page 74). In its most severe form this can cause blindness. According to Anthony Kaiser, Neonatologist at St Thomas' Hospital in London, ROP affects around one third of babies born before 28 weeks. Eight out of ten babies who develop the condition do so only mildly and it sorts itself out with no treatment at all.

The commonest problems are far less serious. They include a mild to moderate squint, and short- or long-sightedness which can be corrected with the right pair of glasses.

Action All premature babies should be examined by an ophthalmologist, preferably before they leave the SCBU to go home, or at any rate when they are around six weeks old, and at regular intervals after that until the blood vessels of their eyes have matured. If there are any signs of ROP they can be watched closely, and if necessary treated with gentle laser therapy. In some health authorities, your baby will also routinely have sight checks for squints, short sight and long sight when he is a year old.

Hearing

Some studies suggest that more than 1 in 10 premature babies (about 13 per cent) may have some form of hearing loss, compared with 1 in 50 babies born at term. Hearing problems are more likely if babies were born extremely prematurely, because their hearing systems are still maturing as late as 24–26 weeks and might still be especially vulnerable to damage if they have to complete the process outside the protection of the womb.

One possible additional cause of hearing damage in premature babies is the surprising amount of noise they are exposed to in the SCBU. Research suggests an incubator can be a very noisy place, with sound levels reaching between 50 and 90 decibels (dB). In an ordinary home, the level is nearer 40 dB. Other risk factors include IVH, shortage of oxygen at birth, severe jaundice, some infections including bacterial meningitis, and a birth weight of less than 1,500g (3lb 5oz).

'Overall, premature babies tend to grow up to be fairly slim and light in their earlier years.

It is normal for their growth to be between the 10th and 25th centile [division or band] on the growth chart; whereas the average term baby's growth is usually somewhere near the middle on the 50th centile.

But, as teenagers, they usually finish up only about an inch shorter than you would have expected them to be by looking at their parents' heights.'

Neil Marlow, Professor of Neonatal Medicine, Nottingham University

Born at 27 weeks, Emily Grace is now a bright and healthy three-year-old, the only remaining signs of her prematurity a degree of long-sightedness easily corrected with glasses, and a squint which will be cured by an operation when she is a little older.

Breathing

Please see *Time to go home*, pages 168–70 on possible breathing problems and coming home with oxygen.

Language abilities

Ideally, a toddler needs to be able to:

★ Respond to simple instructions ('Please give me the ball', or 'Come over here to me') by the time he is about 18 months corrected age.

★ Put two words together by about two years corrected age.

★ Speak a few words which someone who didn't know the child could understand by about two and a half years corrected age.

★ Speak in simple sentences of more than two or three words by the time he is about three.

Action Hearing difficulties can make it harder for a child not only to listen to language but also to speak clearly himself, so it can have a knock-on effect on learning and behaviour. If they cannot hear properly, children may become thoroughly discouraged and so withdraw. They may also appear to be disobedient, or behave aggressively or disruptively out of sheer frustration, so it vital to detect any hearing difficulties as early as possible.

If a baby was born prematurely, especially if he has any of the above risk factors, he needs to be screened by an audiologist before he goes home from the SCBU, then again three to six months later. This will help make sure that, if there is a problem of any sort, it will be diagnosed early, then treated promptly and effectively.

Speech

At around the age of two, as many as 20 to 40 per cent of toddlers who were born prematurely, especially those born at less than 1,000g (2lb 3oz), may have some difficulty with language. If they do have a language problem they often find it easier to understand what is said to them than they do to express themselves with words.

These children usually have normal or above average IQs, so this difficulty with language is not something which is directly linked with their intelligence.

Action It is enormously helful to talk to your child a great deal from the very beginning, even if you think he is too young to understand. Keep an eye on the way your toddler communicates with you, whether he is trying to imitate words, and whether he is succeeding with any, and if you have any concerns at all, let your follow up clinic know. They can always refer your child for a check-up (and for extra help if it is needed) with a specialist speech and language therapist.

Movement

It is fairly common for babies who were born prematurely to have a degree of 'unusual muscle tone' for their first year or so of life. In fact, at least 40 per cent – and possibly as much as 80 per cent – of those born weighing less than 1,600g (3½lb) have this to some extent. Their leg or arm muscles may be stiffer or floppier than usual, their movements may be a bit jerky, and they may have exaggerated or muted muscle reflexes too. However, these things generally sort themselves out without any treatment at all by the time the children are 12–18 months old.

For some infants however, the abnormal muscle tone does not sort itself out and they may be diagnosed as having a degree of cerebral palsy (CP). Doctors define this as 'abnormal posture or movement which has been caused by damage to part of the brain'. In practice, this may mean that a person's muscles are very stiff or even in spasm, which can be painful, or they may be very floppy. Both muscle stiffness and floppiness make it hard to sit, stand, walk or control movement.

Risk factors which make it more likely that a baby may have cerebral palsy include: shortage of oxygen in the womb, at birth or for the first few days afterwards; being born very prematurely; and severe IVH. The type of difficulties a child experiences if he has CP may depend on which area of his brain was damaged, and how mild or severe that damage is.

What parents may notice first Children with cerebral palsy may find it difficult to reach the usual milestones you would expect to see in a baby or toddler's development, such as sitting, crawling, walking and balancing, reaching out for objects, grasping small things and beginning to make smaller and more precise movements, such as colouring and scribbling with crayons. They may also have trouble with their speech, and difficulty eating. Physical symptoms can include joint stiffness, turned out ankles, scoliosis (where the spine leans or twists sideways) or a dislocated hip. Children with cerebral palsy often have IQs which are either normal or above average, but despite this they may experience some learning difficulties too.

Action If your baby is diagnosed as having 'abnormal muscle and/or reflexes' *this does not necessarily mean he has cerebral palsy*. Only three to six per cent of premature babies have true CP and many of these children have only

'Many of the early milestones in a child's development are movement milestones: the age at which they roll over, sit up, crawl, or walk. For many extremely preterm babies these milestones will just arrive late, along with other areas of their development. But most babies do simply catch up later.'

Ros Jones, consultant neonatologist at Wrexham Park Hospital, Slough

Cerebral palsy (CP)

CP can be very mild, moderate or severe. It can also be difficult to diagnose accurately at first. However, the more severely affected a baby is, the more quickly he can be diagnosed, and the more quickly he can be helped (see page 78).

'The doctors said Andy may have cerebral palsy but that they would not be able to tell for sure until he was about a year and a half old. We thought: how can we possibly wait that long to find out? He's a year now, he still has some muscle stiffness but still no one can give us a clear answer. But Andy is a lovely little boy – and what's more, he's ours. We just want to enjoy our son for who he is; we're not going to get obsessed about what might be wrong. We don't want to put a label on him. We'll just see how this all turns out.'

Judith, mother of Andrew, born at 29 weeks

IQ

IQ is one basic and useful measure of intelligence.
'Average intelligence' is considered to be anything over 85 points. Below average (sometimes called below-normal or sub-normal) intelligence is considered to be 70–84 points.

a mild form. What it does mean is that the team at your follow-up clinic will help you monitor his progress until a clearer picture emerges. A physiotherapist or occupational therapist may show you some special gentle exercises for you to help your child do, and other activities to help his muscle and ligament development.

Any observations or changes that mothers and fathers see may provide the most important clues or early warning systems of all. You know your own child best so mention any concerns you have, or any changes you notice.

If your child does have cerebral palsy rather than the type of different muscle tone that disappears after 12–18 months, physiotherapy, regular gentle exercises and stretching can help. Special braces can provide support, and surgery may also, if needed, be used later on to help straighten his limbs.

There is also a good deal of research and experimental work being tried to find other forms of treatment, including using small doses of a substance called botulism toxin. This is a poison, but research at the Walton Centre for Neurology and Neurosurgery in Liverpool suggests that, used carefully, it may relax the painful muscle spasms of cerebral palsy and improve a child's posture and walking, possibly delaying or even in some cases avoiding the need for operations .

For a list of organizations that may be able to help you, please see page 203.

Learning and IQ

The vast majority of children who were born prematurely have a perfectly normal IQ, or an IQ that is above average. Research in the early 1990s found that of very low birthweight premature babies, around two-thirds had IQs of between 85 and 115 (average intelligence). Another quarter (20–24 per cent) had borderline IQs of between 75 and 85 and about one in 20 (5 per cent) had an IQ rating of less than 70.

Babies who were born very prematurely or who had very low birthweights of below 1,000g (2lb 3oz) have a greater risk of having a problem than babies born less prematurely and weighing more than this. Estimates vary, but one large research study found that about one in ten (8–13 per cent) of babies born weighing less than 1,000g had below normal IQ levels. But this also means that nine out of ten of the babies had perfectly normal or even higher than average IQs.

For extremely small premature babies weighing less than 750g (1lb 10oz) at birth, four out of every five had perfectly normal IQ levels, with one in five (20 per cent) having below average IQ.

Action Regular developmental assessment at the hospital follow-up clinic is very important. Keep an eye on your child's progress. If anything worries you at all, or just does not seem quite right, do not let it go. Talk to your health visitor, other mothers of premature babies (they may have

Happy and confident, facing the world

'There are three main factors affecting a baby's IQ. Prematurity, environment and genetics. Babies inherit about 70 per cent of their IQ.'

Neil Marlow, Professor of Neonatal Medicine at Nottingham University

experienced something similar with their own children), your GP or the follow-up clinic.

Try to give your child as much loving support and appropriate stimulation as you can – while still letting him develop at his own pace. This just might not be the same pace as children who were born at term, especially if he has had a difficult start or has a long-term health problem he is trying to cope with or overcome. If you are worried about his progress, ask about the local pre-school teaching support service. They may be able to give you some good ideas about how to help your child's development.

Learning and behaviour

As with other developmental problems, the later a baby was born, the milder and fewer his difficulties are likely to be – but the earlier he was born, the more problems he may have at school.

Starting school Ideally, a school should take your child's corrected age into account, especially if he was born as much as three or four months prematurely (at 24–28 weeks). Your child may not be quite ready to start full-time school at the 'standard' age, particularly if your education authority requires children to join the Reception class when they are four. Unfortunately, not all head teachers may be sympathetic to this idea and, even if they are, they may not be able to help if, as is quite usual, the education authority has strict rules (usually based on funding criteria) about when a child must start. But it is worth asking, because at the very least you may be able to get the head teacher to allow your child just to come for mornings only for a couple of terms if he finds school a bit much to cope with.

Possible problems According to Professor Whitelaw, attention deficit disorder or ADD (short concentration span, impulsiveness) and hyperactivity are about four to five times more common for babies who were born weighing less than 1,500g (3lb 5oz). In any group of small boys and girls, up to 6 per cent might have some degree of either ADD or hyperactivity anyway; however, for children who arrived prematurely some studies put it nearer to 25 per cent.

At the other end of the behavioural spectrum, parents, researchers and teachers also say they have noticed that some children born very prematurely who weighed less than 1,000g (2lb 3oz) at birth are more likely to be quite shy, withdrawn and nervous of being assertive or standing up for themselves at school.

Even when premature children have perfectly normal or above average intelligence ratings – as most do – they also seem to be more likely than term-born children to have difficulties with their school work. Possible problem areas include reading, spelling, maths, abstract reasoning, and difficulty organizing themselves and their work. So extra help at school is still much needed and can make a great deal of difference.

Long-term research which followed up prematurely born children for several years through school up to the ages of nine, ten and eleven has found that there may be 'residual' learning problems. These are difficulties which are not obvious at first, and which are only noticed by parents and teachers as the children become older. The problems may be quite subtle and sometimes go unrecognized for several school years. However, the children tend not to outgrow them on their own, so they may need extra help.

The good news is that only around 10–20 per cent of children who were very low birthweight premature babies and who have normal intelligence have any kind of learning disability which is marked enough for it to affect how they do at school.

Action Understanding, encouragement and support from both parents and teachers is vital. Try to identify any areas in which your child is having difficulty at school as early as possible, ensuring he has special long-term help and support there from the beginning.

If child is fairly quiet, is seen to be getting on with things, makes little fuss, and has no very obvious difficulties with, for example, reading or writing, teachers with big classes to cope with may assume he is doing fine when in fact he may be struggling. This can go on for years before anyone notices.

If you are concerned because you feel your child needs some extra support at school, but his teacher is not convinced, talk to the paediatrician at your child's follow-up clinic. He or she will often be able to support you by writing letters to the school, and referring your child for assessment and help to the right community education support services and officers, such as an educational psychologist.

Regular checks on your child's sight and hearing are important, too, as even minor problems can make a great difference to his understanding of what is going on in the classroom and playground.

As your child gets older (from about four or five) see what outside-school activities he is interested in as these may well help to build up his confidence in himself. Parents often mention that some of the most helpful things for gentle confidence-building include drama, art, music or dance classes, swimming, martial arts, and the special yoga/meditation classes for children that are available in some areas.

If your child does have a learning disorder, whether it is very mild or more serious, it's well worth contacting a parent and family support group (see page 203). These organizations can offer all sorts of help, including moral support and information about everything from the type of diet and nutritional supplements which may help, to special forms of education and how to get educational back-up.

PREMATURE BIRTH: WHY DOES IT HAPPEN?

Perhaps one of the hardest things about having a premature baby is that in one case out of every two, no one can even tell you why it happened. However, parents do often wonder whether there was any reason for their child's early birth, or whether there is any treatment the doctors could give, or some steps they can take for themselves, that might help prevent another premature birth next time.

It's not your fault

Many women feel that if they have a premature baby it must somehow be their fault. Experts say that is very rarely true. On the contrary, they say that women who give birth early have usually done a terrific job of protecting and nurturing their babies under very difficult circumstances.

REASONS FOR PREMATURITY

There are two ways in which babies may be born too soon. One is if their mothers go into labour too early. This is called *premature labour*. Or, there may be a medical problem threatening the well-being of the unborn baby, her mother or sometimes both, and the obstetrician may arrange to deliver the baby early. This is called *premature delivery*.

Causes of premature labour

There are many different reasons for giving birth early, several of which are inter-related. The main causes seem to be:

* **An infection** around the cervix, or in the womb. Other infections, notably those of the kidneys and urinary systems, are also sometimes associated with early labour.

* **A sensitive womb** that can easily be provoked to contract strongly and much earlier than normal, especially if over-stretched by a big baby or twins or more.

* **Other problems with the womb**, such as placental abruption (when the placenta begins to peel away from the womb wall). If there is any bleeding from behind the placenta this may irritate the muscle of the womb and cause early contractions.

* **A weak cervix**, not strong enough to stay closed against the baby's increasing weight.

* **The baby not growing properly**, often because the placenta is not able to transmit enough food and oxygen. Pre-eclampsia (see below) can be a major cause of this.

* **Amniotic sac membranes that begin to weaken or give way early** (your waters breaking early).

* **Carrying twins, triplets or more** can stretch the womb more than just one baby, and it also means extra weight is pressing down on the cervix, which may make it harder for it to remain shut.

* **An unusually shaped womb; or a womb which has a fibroid or fibroids** growing on its walls. Fibroids are benign, non-cancerous whorls of tissue.

* **Too much fluid in the amniotic sac** can put extra pressure on the womb walls and perhaps the cervix too.

* **An abnormality in the fetus.** The mother's body may recognize that an unborn fetus is not developing normally and end the pregnancy by going into early labour. This usually happens in the first 12 weeks, as a miscarriage, but occasionally it may occur later, as a premature birth.

* **Physical trauma**, such as an accident, fall, violence or injury to the woman's belly.

* **Rogue antibodies** that cause blood

clotting in the system. The condition is called thrombophilia.

• 'Placental clock' theory Recent Australian research suggests that If unborn babies are not getting enough food and oxygen, they may be pre-programmed with a survival instinct that causes them to trigger labour – on the grounds that they might be 'better out than in'.

Other causes

There are many, and several of them are inter-related. Yet, as James McGregor, Professor of Obstetrics and Gynaecology at Colorado University, says: 'Premature birth is like heart disease in a way – there are so many different risk factors. And why is it that some mothers with major risk factors don't have their babies prematurely, yet others, with no major risk factors that we can see, do? We still have no idea.'

• **Having diabetes** – or developing it temporarily while you are pregnant. Diabetes is a risk factor for developing pre-eclampsia. So are other long-term health problems such as high blood pressure, and kidney disease.

• **Smoking cigarettes.**

• **Continuously high stress levels.**

• **Being poor.**

• **Heavy drinking** and/or binge drinking.

• **Heavy physical work**, constant standing, heavy lifting, and so on.

• **Taking illegal recreational drugs.** For instance, if you smoke cannabis regularly, research suggests you are more likely to have a low-birthweight baby (low-birth-weight babies have many of the same difficulties as premature babies); cocaine and crack may also be risk factors for having a premature baby, partly because

they cause blood pressure swings, which may encourage placental abruption.

• **Being an underweight mother.**

• **Being an 'older' mother (over 35) or a much younger one (under 17).** It is possible that as you get older, if you do develop pre-eclampsia you may do so more severely. You may also be likely to develop temporary (gestational) diabetes.

• **Infections** causing very high temperatures can trigger premature labour.

• **Becoming pregnant through assisted conception techniques** such as IVF may be a risk factor in so far as it makes multiple pregnancy more likely. However, it tends to be older women who have this type of fertility treatment, and their likelihood of a premature baby may be higher anyway.

• **Work.** There is no proof that working, as such, when you are pregnant makes you more likely to have a premature baby. However, according to a large European study (EUROPOP '98), in addition to heavy manual labour, there are some particular types or aspects of work that may make a difference. These include: jobs that cause continual stress; working long hours with VDUs; and simply working long hours (43 hours or more a week).

Premature delivery

There are various reasons why your doctors may decide it is safest to deliver your baby early.

• **Pre-eclampsia**, a pregnancy-related form of high blood pressure (*note*: raised blood pressure in pregnancy is not uncommon and does not, by itself, mean you have pre-eclampsia). Symptoms include headaches and swelling or puffiness in your hands, feet, legs and sometimes face. It can be detected by regular antenatal checks: signs include raised blood-pressure readings and protein traces in the urine. Pre-eclampsia is most common in first pregnancies, is usually mild, but about one in every hundred women who develop it do so severely. It starts in the placenta, reducing the mother's blood flow and so cutting back the baby's source of nutrition and oxygen. This means the baby will not grow so well, or stop growing altogether or, in extreme cases, may die.

• **Problems with the placenta** can mean your unborn baby is undernourished and not growing properly, so your doctors may feel it would be better if she were delivered early and given the best possible care, and nutrition, on the SBCU. Other problems include placenta praevia (where the placenta is blocking the baby's exit route).

• **Carrying twins, triplets or more.** Your doctors may decide it is safer to deliver them early if perhaps one, or more, of them does not seem to be growing in the womb, or if you are finding being pregnant with more than one baby very difficult.

• **'Maternal reasons'** means that the mother needs an early delivery as she is unable to cope with the pregnancy any longer. For example, she may have severe pain because her pubic bones have separated or may have had troubled previous pregnancies, or a previous pregnancy that ended in stillbirth.

WHAT ABOUT NEXT TIME?

If you have had one premature baby, it is true that you are more likely than a mother whose last baby arrived at term to have another. However, doctors will monitor both your own and your baby's health more closely than the first time around so that they can identify and help treat any problems fast and effectively.

What can you do?

If you are a smoker, try your very best to stop before you become pregnant again, or at the very least, as soon as you know you are pregnant (see page 203 for sources of help and support). Smoking when you are pregnant means that your baby may be born earlier – but it also means that your baby will almost certainly be born smaller, because smoking restricts the food and oxygen she gets in the womb, and retards growth, so she will be more likely to be low birthweight and have many of the same difficulties as premature babies.

If you are taking illegal drugs, try to get as much help as you can to give them up, if possible before you become pregnant again (see page 203 for sources of help).

Try to cut down your stress levels in any way you can, and eat and drink as healthily as possible. Some doctors recommend cutting out alcohol altogether; however, there is some evidence that a single glass of red wine a day may do no harm, as red wine contains ingredients that help prevent blood vessels, including those in the placenta, from damage.

If you had your baby early last time and no one knows why, it is worth asking your hospital to do a simple swab test to check for an infection in your vagina or cervix. Infections in the cervix can be low level, produce no symptoms, live undetected for many years yet still be an important cause of premature labour.

Preventing premature birth

• **Pre-eclampsia**. If you had pre-eclampsia last time, especially if it began before you were 32 weeks pregnant, your doctors may suggest a daily low dose of aspirin (usually 75mg or a quarter of a single adult tablet), beginning when you are about 12 weeks pregnant. Aspirin reduces the blood-clotting chemicals your body makes, and might also discourage your blood vessels from contracting. However, low-dose aspirin is not a self-help treatment: it needs to be taken under the supervision of a hospital consultant.

You will be given frequent and detailed antenatal check-ups throughout your pregnancy to look out for any signs of pre-eclampsia beginning again. These include urine and blood-pressure checks, scans to track your baby's growth and Doppler scans to check the blood flow through the placenta. The hospital may advise bed rest, and might give you medication to keep your blood pressure down. If the pre-eclampsia is making you ill, or it looks as if you may be going into premature labour, you will be admitted to hospital for careful monitoring, bed rest, and possibly drugs to lower your blood pressure.

Recent research at Guys and St Thomas' Hospital in London suggests that vitamins C and E taken in the last half of your pregnancy can help prevent pre-eclampsia developing.

• **Weak cervix**. A surgical stitch may help keep the cervix closed: a study by the Royal College of Gynaecologists found it could work for anything between 1 and 19 weeks, and seemed to help in 50% of cases.

• **Thrombophilia** is relatively rare, though it is more common for women who have an auto-immune disorder called lupus. It can be treated with medications which reduce blood clotting.

• **When the baby is not growing properly**. If this is due to high blood pressure you will be offered drugs to lower it, advised to rest in bed (perhaps in hospital) and be carefully monitored. If your baby's growth seems very restricted, and/or she seems to be in distress, your obstetrician may decide to deliver her and give her the best possible care in the NICU.

Treatments for premature labour

If you are in premature labour already, or if your waters have broken but you have no contractions yet, you may be given anti-biotics to treat existing infections or prevent one developing. This treatment is still experimental, but it may help because it is thought that infections produce in-flammatory substances that trigger labour.

When labour has started

You will be admitted to hospital, monitored carefully, given bed rest and probably offered a drug treatment that can delay premature labour, because unless your baby is in distress (perhaps she is short of oxygen, now) every extra day she spends inside you counts.

A couple of extra days or so make the most difference at around the 26–27 week mark when, American research suggests, an unborn baby is maturing especially fast and her chances of survival rise by around 1 per cent for every extra 24 hours she is able to spend in the womb. Buying a further 24–48 hours also gives your obstetrician vital time to make sure that there is a guaranteed place waiting for her in a good neonatal care unit as soon as she arrives.

Research, medical studies, and resources

EFFECTS OF PREMATURITY;
CARE OF AND INTERACTION
WITH PREMATURE BABIES

Type of handling your baby has
Guidelines for Perinatal Care,
published by the American
Academy of Pediatrics, (1992)
Werner and Conway, 'Caregiver
contacts experienced by
premature infants in neonatal
intensive care', *Maternal-Child
Nursing Journal,* 19:11 (1990),
21–43

Lighting levels in SCBUs
Robinson *et al.,* 'Illuminance of
neonatal units', *Archives of
Diseases in Childhood,* 65 (1990),
679–682
Glass *et al.,* 'Effect of bright light
in the hospital nursery on the
incidence of retinopathy of
prematurity', *New England
Journal of Medicine,* 313:7
(1985), 401–404
J.M. Oehler, 'Developmental care
of low birthweight infants',
Nursing Clinics of North America,
28:2 (1993), 289–301
Lotas, 'Effects of light & sound
in the neonatal intensive care
unit environment in the low
birth weight infant', *Clinical
Issues in Perinatal and Women's
Health Nursing,* 3:1 (1992), 34–44
Treas, 'Incubator covers: health
or hazard?', *Neonatal Network,*
12:8 (1993), 50–51
Whitley and Cowan,
'Developmental intervention in
the newborn intensive care unit',
in NAACO's *Clinical Issues in
Perinatal and Women's Health
Nursing* 2:1 (1991), 84–110

**Babies sleeping only for brief
periods**
S.B. Korones, 'Disturbance and
infants' rest', in T.D. Moore (ed.),
*Report on the 69th Ross
Conference on Pediatric Research,*
Columbus, Ross Laboratories
(1976)

Premature baby massage
T.M. Field, 'Tactile/kinaesthetic
stimulation effects on preterm
neonates', *Pediatrics,* 77 (1986),
654–658
'Effect of touch on the immune
system' in N. Gunzenhauser
(ed.), *Advances in Touch,* Johnson
& Johnson *Paediatric Round
Table,* 1989 14, 22031
C. Kuhn *et al.,*
'Tactile/kinaesthetic stimulation
effects on sympathetic and
adrenocortical function in
preterm infants', *Journal of
Pediatrics,* (1991), 119

Therapeutic touch
A. Carruthers, 'Therapeutic
touch: a force to promote
bonding and wellbeing',
Professional Nurse, (Feb. 1992)
B. Daley, 'Therapeutic touch:
nursing practice and
contemporary cutaneous wound
healing research', *Journal of
Advanced Nursing,* 25,
1123–1132
R.B. Fedoruk, 'Therapeutic touch
as a method for reduction of
stress in premature neonates',
Dissertation in *Abstracts
International,* 46 (1984)
M. Olsen *et al.,* 'Stress induced
immunosuppression and
therapeutic touch', *Alternative
Therapies,* 3:2 (1997), 68–74
J.F. Quinn, 'Transfer of the
relaxation response' (Doctoral
dissertation, University of
Maryland). Also in *The Journal of
Holistic Nursing* 6:1 (1988)
'Therapeutic touch and post-
operative pain: a Rogerian
research study', *Nursing Science
Quarterly,* 6:2

Positioning of baby
C. Amiel-Tyson and A. Grenier,
*Neurological assessment in the
first year of life* (New York,
Oxford University Press, 1986)
Susan Blackburn, 'Problems of

preterm infants after discharge',
JOGNN, (Jan. 1995)
M. Hallsworth, 'Positioning of
the preterm infant', *Paediatric
Nursing,* 7:1 (1995), 18–20
S. Turrill and M. Stein,
'Supported positioning in
intensive care', *Paediatric
Nursing,* 4:4 (1992)
J. Young, 'Nursing preterm
babies in intensive care. Which
position is best?', *Journal of
Neonatal Nursing,* 1:1 (1994)

**Position premature babies lie in
affecting their postural
development**
M. Hallsworth, 'Positioning in
the preterm infant', *Paediatric
Nursing* 7:1 (1995), 18–20
J. Young, 'Nursing preterm
babies in intensive care; which
position is best?', *Journal of
Neonatal Nursing,* 1:1 (1994),
27–31

Positioning/less medication
K.M. Jorgensen, *Developmental
Care of the Premature Infant: A
Concise Overview* (USA, S.
Weymouth, Developmental Care
Division of Children's Medical
Ventures, 1993)
G.B. Merenstein and S.L.
Gardner, *The Handbook of
Neonatal Intensive Care,* (3rd
edition, St Louis, Mosby Year
Book)

Kangaroo care
R.B. Hosseini *et al.,* 'Pre-term
infants and fathers:
psychological and behavioural
effects of skin-to-skin contact',
Ursus Medicus, 2 (1992), 47–55
Susan Ludington-Hoe with
Susan K. Golant, *Kangaroo Care:
The Best You Can Do To Help Your
Preterm Infant* (Bantam, 1996)
Susan Ludington-Hoe and G.C.
Anderson, 'Preliminary results of
very early kangaroo care for
preterm infants', paper presented
at 8th National Meeting of the

Nurses Association of the American College of Obstetricians & Gynaecologists, Orlando, 1991

Susan Ludington-Hoe and F. Hashemia, 'Temporal relationship between kangaroo care and crying', paper presented at the International Sigma Theta Tau Meeting, November 1991

C. Virgin, 'The kangaroo method brings the child back to its mother', *Sygeplejersken* 11 (1987)

Whitelaw et al., 'Skin to skin contact for very low birthweight infants and their mothers: a randomized trial of kangaroo care', *Archives of Diseases in Childhood* 63 (1988), 1377–81

Born smiling

Frederick Leboyer, *Birth Without Violence* (Cedar Press, 1995)

Doing what, when: term and preterm babies

Joan Gomez, *Childhood Development*, (Vermilion, 1997)

Frank Manginello and Theresa Foy DiGeronimo, *Your Premature Baby*, (USA, John Wiley, 1991)

Joseph J. Volpe, *Neurology of the New-born* (2nd edition, Philadelphia, W.B. Saunders, 1987), 73–74

Premature survival rates

Tin et al., 'Changing prognosis for babies of less than 28 weeks gestation', *British Medical Journal* 1997, 314

J. Morrison, 'Clinical, scientific and ethical aspects of fetal and neonatal care at extremely preterm periods of gestation', *British Journal of Obstetrics & Gynaecology*, 104 (Dec. 1997), 1341–1350

Unborn babies, awareness in womb

Nikki Bradford, *The Miraculous World of Your Unborn Baby* (Bramley Books, 1998)

Busnel et al., 'Fetal audition', *Annals of New York Academy of Sciences*, 662 (1992), 118–134

David Chamberlain, *The Mind of Your Newborn Baby* (North Atlantic Books, 1998)

E. Stenneert et al., 'Incubator noise and hearing loss', *Early Human Development* 1:1,

113–115

Van de Carr et al., 'Effects of a prenatal intervention programme', in Feydor-Freyburgh and M. Vogel (ed.), *Prenatal & Perinatal Psychology & Medicine – A Comprehensive Survey of Research & Practice*, (Parthenon Publications, 1988)

Van de Carr, R. and M. Lehrer, *The Prenatal Classroom – a Parents Guide to Teaching Your Baby in the Womb* (Atlanta, Humanics Learning, 1992)

Zimmer et al., 'Response of premature fetus to stimulation by speech sounds', *Early Human Development*, 33, 207–215

Individualized premature baby care programmes

H. Als, 'A synactive model of neonatal behaviour organisation: a framework for the assessment of neurobehavioral development in the premature infant', *Physical & Occupational Therapy in Paediatrics*, 6 (1986), 3–53

H. Als, Duffy et al., 'Earliest intervention for preterm infants in the newborn intensive care unit', in M. J. Guralnick (ed.), *The Effectiveness of Early Intervention* (Baltimore Books), 47–76

S.K. Collins and K. Kuck, 'Music therapy in the neonatal intensive care unit', *Neonatal Network*, 9:6 (1991), 23–26

Dossey, Keegan, Guzzetta, Kilkmeyer, *Holistic Nursing: A Handbook for Practice*, (1995)

Richard Gerber, *Vibrational Medicine* (Santa Fe, Bean & Co., 1988)

H. Als et al., 'Individualised behavioural and environmental care for the vlbw preterm infant at high risk for BPD: NICU and developmental outcome', *Paediatrics* 78:6 (1986), 1123–1132

H. Als et al., 'Individualised behavioural and environmental care for the vlbw preterm infant at high risk of BDP and IVH, study II: NICU Outcome', Abstract, New England Perinatal Association, Woodstock, Vermont, 1988

H. Als, G. Lawhon, F.H. Duffy et al., 'Individualised behavioural and environmental care of the VLBW infant at high risk for bronchopulmonary dysplasia and intraventricular haemorrhage', *Journal of the American Medical Association*, 272(11) (1994)

A. Kleberg, B. Westrup et al., 'Evaluation of the newborn individualised developmental care & assessment program (NIDCAP) in a Swedish setting', *Perinatal & Neonatal Medicine*, 1997

P. Petryshen et al., 'Comparing nursing costs for preterm infants receiving conventional vs developmental care', *Nursing Economics*, 15:3 (1997)

S. Whitley and M. Cowan, 'Developmental intervention in newborn and intensive care unit', *Clinical Issues on Perinatal and Women's Health Nursing*, 2:11 (1991), 84–110

Feeding

'Human milk and the pre-term baby', *Lancet*, 306 (1993), 1628–1629

'Cure in mothers' milk', *New Scientist*, April 20, 1991

'The quality of a mother's milk and the health of her child; beliefs and practices of the women of Mithilia', *Soc. Sci. Med.* 27, 461–469

S.J. Gross et al., 'Nutritional composition of milk produced by mothers delivering preterm', *Journal of Pediatrics*, 1980

N.B. Mathur et al., 'Anti-infective factors in preterm human colostrum', *Acta Paediatrica Scandinavica*, 79, 1039–44

G.C. McCain, 'Promotion of preterm infant nipple feeding with non-nutrative sucking', *Journal of Pediatric Nursing*, 10:1 (1995), 3–8

Sandra Lang, *Breastfeeding Special Care Babies* (Bailliere Tindall, 1997)

C.S. Shaker, 'Nipple Feeding Premature Infants: A Different Perspective', *Neonatal Network*, 1990

P.A. Steer et al., *Effective Care of the Newborn Infant*, Sinclair and Bracken (ed.), (Oxford

University Press, 1992)
A. Whitelaw, G. Heisterkamp, K. Sleath et al., 'Skin to skin contact for very low birthweight infants and their mothers; a randomized trial of kangaroo care', Archives of Diseases in Childhood, 63 (1988)

Cues
S.T. Blackburn and K.A. Vandenburg, 'Assessment and management of neonatal neurobehavioral development', in Comprehensive Neonatal Nursing: A Physiological Perspective (Philadelphia, W.B. Saunders, 1993), 1094–1133
Bernadette Carter, 'Pantomimes of pain, distress, repose and lability: the world of the pre-term baby', Journal of Child Health Care, 1 (Spring 1997)
P.K. Hiniker and L. Moreno, Developmentally Supportive Care – Theory and Application (self-study module) (S and S.W. Vickers)
Carly J. Semmler and Sharon Dowling Butcher, Handle With Care: Articles About the At-Risk Neonate (Tucson, Therapy Skill Builders, 1990)
Kathleen A. Vandenberg and Linda S. Franck, 'Behavioural issues for infants with BPD', Neonatal Network 22, (1990)

COMMON PROBLEMS FOR PREMATURE BABIES
Jeanette Zaichkin (ed.), Newborn Intensive Care, (Petaluma, Ca., NICU-LINK Publishers, 1997)
SIDS/Apnoea connection
American Academy of Pediatrics and American College of Obstetricians and Gynaecologists, 'Postpartum and follow-up care' in R.K. Freeman and R.L. Poland (ed.), Guidelines for Perinatal Care (3rd edition, Illinois, American Academy of Pediatrics, 1996)
Time spent not breathing: how common it is
Glotzbach, Baldwin et al., 'Periodic breathing in preterm infants: incidence and characteristic', Pediatrics, 84 (1989), 785–792

Apnoea/bradycardia spells regularly missed in SCUs
Graff, Soriano et al., 'Undetected apnoea and bradycardia in infants in special care units (both term and prem)', Pediatric Pulmonology, 11 (1991), 195–7
Bradycardia
A. Hodgman et al., 'Episodes of bradycardia during early infancy in the term born and pre term infant', Journal of Diseases of Childhood, 147 (1993), 960–964
Baby monitors
J. Levine et al., at the Mayo Clinic, Rochester, Minnesota in Science, (Jan. 1999) Report on baby monitors in Which? Magazine, volume 4 (Feb. 1996)
J. Levine et al., Report by FSID, (Nov. 1999)
The National Advisory Board's 3rd Annual Confidential Enquiry into stillbirths and deaths in infancy, 1996
Humidity for premature babies with dry, fragile skin
Ann Marshall, 'Humidifying the environment for the premature neonate', Journal of Neonatal Nursing, (Jan. 1977)
Jaundice
S. Edward, 'Providing safe care for jaundiced infants', Phototherapy and the Neonate, (Oct. 1995)
Protecting skull of very low birthweight baby from pressure induced IVF
J. Dietch, 'Periventricular-intraventricular haemorrhage in the VLBW infant', Neonatal Network, 12.1 (1993)
'Neurological Assessment of the Preterm and Full Term Infant', SIMP Clinical Developmental Medicine 79, L. and V. Dubowitz (ed.), 1979

MORE SERIOUS PROBLEMS
Debbie Fraser Askin, 'Major medical problems' in Jeanette Zaichkin (ed.), Newborn Intensive Care – What Every Parent Needs to Know', (Petaluma Ca., NICU-LINK Publishers, 1997)
Henry Halliday, 'Surfactant therapy: questions and answers',

Journal of Neonatal Nursing, (May 1997)
M. Rowe, 'Asphyxiated infants', Neonatal Network, 9:4, 7–10
Robinson (ed.), Textbook of Neonatology (New York, Churchill Livingstone)
IVH
'Periventricular-intraventricular haemorrhage in the very low birthweight infant', Neonatal Network 12:11, 7–16
Anthony Kaiser, IVH parents' information leaflet, St Thomas' Hospital, London
Eyesight
K.M. Gracey and K.L. McLaughlin, 'Caring for the infant with retinopathy of prematurity undergoing cryotherapy', Neonatal Network, 9:7 (1991), 7–12
Lighting
J.M. Oehler, 'Developmental care of low birth weight infants', Nursing Clinics of North America, 28:2 (1993), 209–301
M. Gordon Shogan and L.L. Schumann, 'The effect of environmental lighting on the oxygen saturation of preterm infants in the NICU', Neonatal Network, 12:5 (1993), 7–13
BDP
John Loftus, 'Medical matters: mechanical ventilation of babies', Newborn News, (Autumn 1992)
Sedatives making some babies more sensitive to pain
R.J. Roberts, Drug Therapy in Infants: Pharmacologic Principles and Clinical Experienc (Philadelphia, W.B. Saunders, 1984)
Katherine A. Vandenberg and Linda S. Frank, 'Behavioural issues for infants with BPD', Neonatal Network, 1990

MOTHERS
Tilly Padden and Sheila Glenn, 'Maternal experiences of preterm birth and neonatal intensive care', Journal of Reproductive and Infant Psychology, 15 (1997), 121–139
Caesarean statistics: 1998 provisional figures available from the Information and Statistics

Division of the Common Services Agency for the National Health Service in Scotland

THE PREMATURE BABY AT HOME
Premature babies' behaviour after they leave SCBU
Susan Berger et al., 'Caring for the graduate from the neonatal unit: at home, in the office, and in the community', *Pediatric Clinics of North America*, 45:3 (June 1998)
'Fostering family developmental after preterm hospitalisation' in R.A. Ballard (ed.) *'Pediatric Care of the NICU Graduate'* (Philadelphia, W.B. Saunders, 1988)
Ways in which preterm babies' brains and nervous systems develop differently/at different pace from term babies'
'Structural and neurobehavioral delay in postnatal brain development of preterm infants', *Pediatric Resources*, 39 (1996), 895–901
Weaning
Caroline King, 'Weaning preterm infants onto solids: when, why and how', *The Journal of Neonatal Nursing*. 4:6 (1998)
Martinez-Augustine et al., 'Dietary nucleotides might influence the humoral immune response against cow's milk protein in preterm neonates', *Biology of the Neonate*, 71 (1997), 215–23
Possible problems areas and their solutions
Susan Blackburn, 'Problems of preterm infants after discharge', JOGNN, (Jan. 1995)
L. Termini et al., 'Reasons for acute care visits and re-hospitalization in VLBW infants', *Neonatal Network* 8 (1990), 23–26

PREMATURE BABIES: OUTCOMES AND DEVELOPMENT IN THE FIRST FEW YEARS
General
'The EPICure Study – summary and results', steering group: P. Steer, K. Costeloe, A. Gibson, I. Laing, M. Lewins, N. Marlow, P.

Pharoah, A. Wilkinson (April 1999)
Susan Blackburn, 'Problems of preterm infants after discharge', *JOGNN*, (Jan. 1995)
Hack et al., 'Long term developmental outcomes of low birthweight infants', *The Future of Children*, 5:1 (Spring 1995)
Supporting parents of very preterm children
Neil Marlow et al., 'Randomised trial of parental support for families of very preterm children', *Archives of Diseases of Childhood Fetal Neonatal Ed*, 79 (1998), 4–11
Bright lighting possibly affecting vision: see above, 'How Being Born Early Can Affect Your Baby', particularly Glass (1985), Oehler (1993), Lotas (1992) and Janine Young, *Developmental Care of the Premature Baby* (Balliere Tindall, 1996)
Noise in SCBUs possibly affecting hearing
M.D. Letko, 'Detecting and preventing infant hearing loss', *Neonatal Network*, 1992
'Developmental care of low birth weight infants', *Nursing Clinics of America*, 1993 28:2 (1993), 289–301
K.M. Jorgensen, *Developmental Care of the Premature Infant: A Precise Overview* (Children's Medical Ventures, 1993)
Growth
J.L. Manser, 'Growth in the high risk neonate', *Clinics in Perinatology*, 11 (1984), 19–40
IQ levels
G. Escobar, B. Littenberg et al., 'Outcome among surviving very low birthweight infants; a meta analysis', *Archives of Diseases in Childhood* 66 (1991), 201–211
Hearing
Hack et al., 1993, see above
Sight
S.W. Teplin et al., 'Neurodevelopment health and growth status at age 6 years of children with birth weight of less than 1,00lg', *Journal of Pediatrics*, 118 (1991), 768–777

Learning problems at school
S.T. Bernbaum and M. Hoffman-Williamson, *Primary Care of the Preterm Infant* (St Louis, Mosby Year Book, 1991)
M. Ornstein, Ohlsson et al., 'Neonatal follow-up of low birthweight/extremely low birthweight infants to school age: a critical overview', *Acta Paediatrica Scandinavica*, 80 (1991), 741–748
S. Saigal et al., 'Intellectual and functional status at school entry of children who weighed 1,000g or less at birth; a regional perspective of birth in the 1980s', *Journal of Pediatrics*, 116 (1990), 409–416

PREMATURITY: CAUSES AND FUTURE PREVENTION
J. Morrison, 'Clinical, scientific and ethical aspects of fetal and neonatal care at extremely preterm periods of gestation', *British Journal of Obstetrics & Gynaecology* 104 (Dec. 1997)
Cervical stitches
J.M. Aarts et al., 'Emergency cervical cerclage', Obstetrics 7 Gynaecology survey 50, 1995
J. MacDougall et al., 'Emergency cervical cerclage', *British Journal of Obstetrics & Gynaecology*, 98 (1991)
Antibiotics
J.C. Hauth et al., 'Reduced incidence of preterm delivery with metronidazole and erythromycin in women with bacterial vaginosis', *New England Journal of Medicine* 333 (1995)
Ritrodine
Canadian Preterm Labour Investigators group, 'Treatment of preterm labour with the beta-adrenergic agonist ritrodine', *New England Journal of Medicine* 327 (1992)
Corticosteroids
P. Crowley, 'Corticosteroids prior to preterm delivery', in M.W. Enkin et al., *Pregnancy & Childbirth Module of The Cochrane Database of Systematic Reviews*, updated Sept. 1996

Effects of mother's stress levels on baby
L. Ellis and W. Peckham 'Prenatal stress and left-handedness among offspring', *International Journal of Pre and Perinatal Psychology and Medicine*, (Winter 1991), 135–143
V. Glover *et al.*, 'Association between maternal anxiety during pregnancy and increased uterine artery resistance index: cohort based study', *British Medical Journal* 318:7177 (Jan. 6, 1999), 153–7
Hans Lou, 'How prenatal stressors for the mother affect foetal brain development', Proceedings published from the bi-annual meeting of the Marce Society, London 1996
B.R.H. Van den Bergh, 'The influence of maternal emotions during pregnancy on fetal – and neonatal – behaviour', *The International Journal of Pre and Perinatal Psychology and Medicine* (Winter 1990)
A.J. War, 'Stress and childhood psychopathology', *Child Psychiatry and Human Development* 22 (1991), 97–110
Nikki Bradford, *The Miraculous World of your Unborn Baby*, Salamander (2000)
Placental clock/CRH contractions
R. Smith, 'Alterations in the hypothalamic pituitary adrenal axis during pregnancy and the placental clock that determines the length of parturition', *Journal of Reproductive Immunology*, 39:1–2 (August 1998), 215–220

GETTING INFORMATION ON THE INTERNET

There is a wealth of information about prematurity on the Net: potential treatments, possible causes, treatments for premature babies themselves, what sort of difficulties they may experience when they are growing up and what can help done to help. There are also details of everything, including premature baby equipment, slings, car seats, clothes and support groups. Some of the most useful *medical* sites include:

Tommy's Campaign http://www.tommys-campaign.org provides information to parents and midwives on pregnancy issues.

MEDLINEplus http://medlineplus.nlm.nih.gov/ Thought up by the US National Library of Medicine, MEDLINEplus, which is part of MEDLINE, the biggest database of medical papers in the world, has a variety of useful resources. They include pre-prepared searches (which mean you don't have to worry about the complexities and quirks of the MEDLINE database, which are many), the latest medical news, even medical dictionaries.

Mining Co http://www.mining.com/ has two useful health sections with clear, jargon-free information. One covers general health, the other specifically women's health. Useful links with alternative medicine sites and support groups.

Health on the Net http://www.hon.ch/ A panel of experts has evaluated the info sites and divides your hits into 'recommended' and 'non-checked', giving info on each to tell you whether the sites are worth visiting or not. Asthma, for example, produces 1,600 unchecked and 64 approved.

Medical World Search http://www.mwsearch.com/ A bit confusing at first as it has several different settings that you can alter. But has a search engine that yields lots of proper published research papers from high quality medical journals, so worth getting used to if it is hard, published clinical info and data you are after.

Medscape http://www.medscape.com/ A site aimed at health professionals with detailed, heavyweight published clinical papers and research. Can give you very useful information if you don't mind the medical terminology.

Healthfinder http://www.healthfinder.org/ This was developed by the US Department of Health & Human Services and helps you find databases, websites, support and self-help groups and on-line publications.

Health Centre – The Clinic http://www.healthcentre.org.uk/hc/clinic/websites/default.htm This has an index to UK health web sites.

NET TIPS

If you are not on-line at work or home, there are cyber cafes springing up countrywide, (which as well serving coffee, have helpful staff to get you started on your Net searches) and many computers linked to the Net in major libraries. You pay as you go for the time you spend on the Net.

Anyone can publish anything on the Net, and they frequently do. So it is worth keeping the following in mind before accepting any info that you find:

• Who is funding this site? Owner's name should be given along with any sponsorship/advertising deals.

• Is the information you are looking at there up to date? A good Web page will say when a piece of info was written, and when it was last updated. Be wary of health pages that don't.

• Interesting article – but does it have a named author? If it is written by someone who says they are an expert in this particular thing, run a search on MEDLINE to see if they have ever had anything on the subject published in a professional peer review journal (i.e. where a relevant panel of experts assesses each article or piece of research before they will use it). If they haven't, or if there doesn't seem to be any author that you can see, be wary.

• Ignore anything offering 'miracle/wonder cures'.

• Or anything which is only backed up by 'delighted customer' testimonials rather than published clinical research carried out by someone *other than* the company selling the product.

CARING FOR YOUR CHILD

Consultant neonatalogist

Senior house officer (SHO)

Consultant paediatrician

Registrar

Nurses

Staff nurses

Chaplain

YOU AND YOUR PREMATURE BABY

Nutritionist

Social worker

Nursery sister

Physiotherapist

Breast-feeding counsellor

Clinical psychologist

Audiologist

IMPORTANT SPECIALIST SUPPORTING PLAYERS

Paediatric radiologist

Paediatric neurologist

Paediatric ophthalmologist

Paediatric cardiologist

Community neonatal nurse

Hospital paediatrician

Follow-up clinic nurses

Occupational therapist

Paediatric neurologist

Genetics department

YOU AND YOUR GROWING CHILD

Portage education

Physiotherapist

Speech therapist

Health visitor

Paediatric ophthalmologist

GP

Paediatric audiologist

Neonatalogist

HELPLINES AND SUPPORT GROUPS

PREMATURITY: WHY DOES IT HAPPEN AND WHAT CAN BE DONE?

APEC (Action on Pre-Eclampsia), 31–33 College Road, Harrow, Middlesex HA1 1EJ Helpline: 020 8427 4217
National charity which supports women with pre-eclampsia. Wide range of information leaflets and booklets, factsheets, newsletter and an Expert Consultation service (list of specialists in pre-eclampsia, recommended by the charity, and with whom they can put you in touch).

Foresight (The Association for the Promotion of Preconceptual Care), 28 The Paddock, Godalming, Surrey GU7 1XD 01483 427 8393
Registered charity which offers both partners detailed guidance on nutrition and detoxification to help them be in the best possible physical health for creating and maintaining a healthy pregnancy. Many of the couples who go to Foresight have a history of miscarriage, infertility, stillbirth and premature birth.

Quitline offers help, support, practical tips, and information for anyone trying to give up smoking. Also has a special counselling service, *Pregnancy Quitline* 0800 00 22 00 for women who are already pregnant and would like to stop smoking, or who are planning to become pregnant and want to give up smoking before they do. The counselling service will call you back six times over a period of time (times/dates of your choosing) to offer you ongoing support.

British Diabetic Association, 10 Queen Anne Street, London W1M 0BD 020 7323 1531
National charity offering wide range of support and information for people with diabetes, including pregnant women who have developed gestational diabetes.

TAMBA (Twins & Multiple Births Association), Harnott House, 309 Chester Road, Little Sutton, Ellesmere Port CH66 1QQ. 0151 348 0020. Twinline: 01732 868 000 7pm–11pm weekdays, 10am–11pm weekends
National support, help and information service for parents who have twins, triplets or more on all aspects of looking after their children from conception to adolescence. Local parents support groups countrywide.

Women's Aid National Helpline, 0345 023 486
Support and information for women experiencing any form of violence or bullying from their partner.

The National Drugs Helpline, 0800 776 600, 24 hours a day, 7 days a week

Free and confidential counselling over the phone. Can also put you in touch with local organizations, support groups and clinics in your area which specialize in helping women who are pregnant (or would like to become pregnant) but are taking illegal drugs, and want to stop.

The British Dietetic Association, 0121 616 4900
Contact the Association for details of nutritionists who have a three-year specialist training recognised by the NHS.

Tommy's Campaign, 1 Kennington Road, London SE1 7RR 020 7620 0188
National pregnancy research charity funding a nationwide programme of research into miscarriage, stillbirth and premature birth. It also provides information to parents and midwives.

WHAT CAN WE DO?

The British Association of Therapeutic Touch, Highland Hall, Renwick, Penrith, Cumbria 01768 898 375

The Osteopathic Centre for Children, 109 Harley Street, London W1N 1DG 020 7486 6160
The organization trains specialist paediatric osteopaths, and may be able to put you in touch with one who has a special interest and experience of working with premature babies, both on the SCBU and afterwards. Also has a charitable clinic for children from 0–18 years, and has an outreach team going regularly to the Starlight Room SCBU, Barnet Hospital, London. See below at *You and your Family* for general osteopathy.

Kangaroo Care
Helpful booklet by Kathy Sleath, the neonatal nursing sister who pioneered kangaroo care in Britain. £2.00 incl. p&p from BLISS (see below at *Time to go home*).

Observing, protecting, comforting, positioning
An excellent book is *Developmental Care of the Premature Baby* by Janine Young, published by Balliere Tindall (1996, currently being updated). Looks at effects of positioning, light, sound, handling etc. Aimed at neonatal staff, but straightforward to read.

Homeopathy
To contact a homeopath who is also a medical doctor call the **British Homeopathic Society** on 020 7935 2163. For a non medically trained professional homeopath contact the Society of Homeopaths on 01604 21400.

Feeding
The National Childbirth Trust, Alexandra House, Oldham Terrace,

London W3 6NH 020 8992 8637
La Leche League of Great Britain, BM 3424, London WC1N 3XX 020 7242 1278. Supports mothers who want to breastfeed.
TAMBA (see above)
CLAPA (The Cleft Lip and Palate Association), 6 Blenheim Close, Danbury, Essex CM3 4NE 01245 225 657
Also has an extension at the Hospital for Sick Children, Great Ormond Street, London WC1N 3JH 020 7405 9200 (main switchboard, ask for the CLAPA extension).

YOU AND YOUR FAMILY

Association for Post Natal-Illness, 25 Jerdan Place, London SW6 1BE 020 7386 0868
According to APNI, mothers who have their babies prematurely run a far higher risk of developing some degree of PNI than mothers who have their babies at full term. This organization is a national charity, and has a network of befrienders (telephone support from other mothers who have recovered from PND). Answers queries by letter on treatments, backed by APNI eminent board of obstetricians and psychiatrists. Can advise on where to get good counselling/treatment. Helpful range of information literature, newsletters.

Caesarean Support Network, c/o Yvonne Williams, 55 Cooil Drive, Douglas, Isle of Man 01624 661269 after 6pm, or at weekends. If writing, please send sae.

The General Osteopathic Council, 020 7357 6655.
Ongoing back pain? The GOC can tell you how to find a professional registered osteopath in your area.

The National Childbirth Trust, Alexandra House, Oldham Terrace, London W3 6NH 020 8992 8637
Homeopathy (see above)

Older brothers and sisters
Special Care Babies by Althea (available from BLISS, £1.50 plus p&p)
An illustrated story for young children about having a premature brother or sister in special care. Includes simple drawings of the neonatal unit and gentle explanations of what happens when a baby is in special care.

TIME TO GO HOME

BLISS, 2nd floor, Camelford House, 87–89 Albert Embankment, London SE1 7PT
020 7820 9471 Helpline support network 0500 618 140, 10am–5pm, Monday–Friday
The main national charity supporting parents of premature babies, and

raising money for vital equipment in neonatal units. Has a regular newsletter, expert medical advisory panel. Also offers a new countrywide network for putting parents in touch with other experienced prem parents. Wide range of information resources including leaflets/info sheets on many aspects of premature baby health and care, books, cassettes, where to find special clothes, nappies, slings, soothers for premature babies.

Clothes and home equipment for premature babies

There are several mail order companies to choose from, including *Little Beginnings* (for babies weighing from 1lb and upwards – they also have a prem baby car seat) on 0116 278 3336; *Small Wonder* (020 8886 1956, clothing only);Tiddlywinks (clothing for babies weighing 2lb upwards) 01274 561 751; *Babycare-Dolly Care (Cosby) Ltd* on 0116 278 3336. Wide range to fit babies from 3lbs upwards. Also the *Incubaby* range for babies weighing 1lb upwards is specially for infants in incubators (designed to accommodate tubing); and *Tiny Trends* on 01202 660 880.

Baby slings suitable for prems – BLISS suggests the Sling Easy, from *Kids in Comfort* 01189 404 942 or the *Wilkinet* Baby Carrier (01239 831 246) suitable for very tiny babies. Nappies for babies weighing 4lbs and upwards can be delivered to your home from Boots' Mother & Baby Direct Line on 0845 840 1000. BLISS also has a good deal of information about specialist companies who supply both clothing (including some from named shops and department stores such as Woolworth's Ladybird range), knitting/sewing patterns, and equipment for premature babies such as teats and comforters. They also have a small collection of donated prem baby clothes which are available under special circumstances – including booties, bonnets, blankets and cardigans.

CRY-SIS, 020 7404 5011
National charity offering confidential support and advice for parents whose babies cry excessively, or sleep poorly.

Parentline, 08088 002 222
Support, counselling and a friendly listening ear for parents who are under stress, and who have children of any age.
See also *TAMBA, NCT, La Leche* (above)

Relate, Head office, 01788 573241, which can put you in touch with your local Relate branch. If the stress of having had a premature baby is telling on your relationship with your partner, you might like to talk to a counsellor.

The Health Information Service (HIS), Freephone 0800 665544 9am–7pm Monday–Thursday, 9am–5pm Friday
Has a large database of nearly all the self-help and support groups in the country classified under the name of the health issue or problem (i.e. if you want to talk to the association which supports parents of autistic children but do not know the organization's name, HIS can find it for you).

The Foundation for the Study of Infant Deaths, 020 7222 8001 9am–5pm
Advice, help, support and information on all aspects of cot death, including what you can do to help prevent it.

SPECIAL BABIES, SPECIAL CHILDREN

SCOPE, Free Helpline 0800 626 216, 9am–9pm weekdays, 2–6pm weekends
The national information and support charity for people of all ages with any degree of cerebral palsy. They have a very wide range of professional support and resources for both parents and children.

National Deaf Children's Society, 15 Dufferin Street, London EC1Y HUR Helpline: 020 7250 0123.
Support, resources, and information for parents whose children have any level of hearing impairment whatsoever, from temporary glue ear and very slight permanent hearing loss upwards.

Royal National Institute for the Blind, Helpline 020 7388 1266
Again, the name is a bit misleading because this national charity has a very wide range of services (books, leaflets, support groups, education programmes, special holidays, advice) for both children and adults whose vision is impaired, whether mildly or severely.

LOOK, (National Federation of Families with Visually Impaired Children) 49 Court Oak Road, Harbourne, Birmingham 0121 428 5038

The Partially Sighted Society, Queens Road, Doncaster DN1 2NX 01302 363852

National Asthma Campaign, Providence House, Providence Place, London N1 ONT 020 7226 2260 Helpline: 0845 7 010 203 9am–7pm
Advice, information and support on all aspects of asthma in adults and children

The Informed Parent, PO Box 870, Harrow, Middlesex HA3 7UW 020 8861 1022
Information service for parents who have any concerns over potential side effects of the standard programme of immunisations for babies and children.

The National Epilepsy Association, National Helpline: 0808 800 5050

The Attention Deficit Family Support Group UK, 01373 826 045
For families with children who have ADD, are hyperactive, or both.

The Hyperactive Children's Support Group, 01903 725 182

National Action and Research for Hyperactivity and ADD, 011628 523 539

The Family Fund, PO Box 5, York YO1 2ZX 01904 621115
Can provide financial help for parents of children with special needs. They are a government funded agency, administered by the Joseph Rowntree Foundation.

Network '81, 1–7 Woodfield Terrace, Stansted, Essex CM24 8AJ 01279 647415
Has an information and advice line for parents of children with special needs, open between 10am and 2pm

The Association for Spina Bifida and Hydrocephalus, ASBAH House, 42 Park Road, Peterborough, Cambridgeshire PE1 2UQ 01733 555 988
See also TAMBA, The National Asthma Campaign, Parentline, Relate, CRY-SIS, and HIS in *Time to go home above.*

GRIEVING AND LOSS

Child Bereavement Trust, Brindley House, 4 Burkes Road, Beaconsfield, Buckinghamshire HP9 1PB 01494 678 088
The trust is a national charity which supports bereaved families whose children have died at any age, and which also offers training/support to professional carers. They have a wide range of clear, sympathetic and highly informative resources especially for parents, including bereavement workshops, books/videos/cassettes for families.

The Foundation for the Study of Infant Deaths, Artillery House, 11–19 Artillery Row, London SW1P 2RT
Have a 24-hour Cot Death Helpline 020 7232 2090 for parents who are either worried about the possibility of cot death, or who have lost a baby in this way.

Stillbirth and Neonatal Death Society, Helpline 0207 436 5881
For parents whose babies were not alive when they were born, or who died when they were still young infants.

See also **Getting Information on the Internet** on page 201

index

Page numbers in *italics* indicate illustrations.

Publishers' acknowledgments

The impulse to produce this book stemmed from the life of a baby who is very special to us: Gianni Litchmore Bonfanti, who was born on 3 July 1997, at 23 weeks, and lived for nine weeks.
Commissioning Editor Jo Christian
Editor Sarah Mitchell
Editorial help Michael Brunström,
                  Judith Warren
Index Tarrant Ranger Indexing

Art Editor Louise Kirby
Designer Becky Clarke
Art Director Caroline Hillier

Production Hazel Kirkman

Photographic acknowledgments

All photographs copyright © Sandra Lousada, except for the following:
© Sam Richards pages 19, 31, 91
© Martin Sharratt pages 58, 103, 139, 143
© Pauline Sharratt page 63
The photograph on page 67 was taken by a nurse in Kingston Hospital.
Sandra Lousada would like to say that, although she took the great majority of the photographs that appear in this book, the two photographs she considers the best were not taken by her or by any professional photographer, but by parents. Sam Richards took the photograph of Ellen on page 19, and Martin Sharratt took the photograph of Isabel and John on page 103; she hopes this will inspire parents to take and value their own pictures of their children.
We are very grateful to all the parents who allowed us to photograph their babies for this book. Special thanks to the parents of: Simone and Amber Eakins, Joseph Edu, Ella and George Ewart, Gabrielle Fulgoni, Elizabeth Hackney, Emily Grace Hale, Tom, Ben and Megan Hughes-Jones, Aaron Jarvis, Ryan Munday, Baby Namwenda, Archie, Storm and Imogen Parrish, George Schiessl, Nina and Ellen Taurich, John Sharratt, Alec Sargood, and Matthew Withington.
We also wish to thank St Thomas' Hospital, London, Kingston Hospital NHS Trust, Surrey and Santa Monica Hospital UCLA, who gave us permission to take photographs in their Special Care Baby Units, and Nurse Bada and Nurse Beverley who allowed us to photograph them.